# Praise for I{

"This is a much-needed book! Teeth are living organs, and their health is closely connected with the health of the whole body. Unhealthy gums, root canals, amalgam fillings, and other dental problems can cause severe degenerative conditions including any autoimmune disease, fibromyalgia, chronic fatigue, multiple sclerosis, allergies, and digestive problems. We need wholistic dentistry more than ever today, and this book is written by a wholistic dentist. I warmly recommend this book!"

**—Dr. Natasha Campbell-McBride**,
author of *Gut and Psychology Syndrome*

"Having grown up in a family in which my father and grandfather were both dentists, I must admit I wanted nothing to do with the subject. Unfortunately for me that meant I have spent most of my career choosing to ignore the profound connection between dental health and whole body health. The concise and informative book by Dr. Nischwitz showed me in very clear terms that this has been a mistake. Many things affect our overall health, but perhaps none are as important as the state of our teeth. I encourage everyone to read *It's All in Your Mouth* and start putting Dr. Nischwitz's ideas into action."

**—Tom Cowan, MD**, author of *Cancer and the New Biology of Water*

"There's been a huge shift in awareness about how to achieve optimal health, but many people still miss where it all begins: the mouth. *It's All in Your Mouth* cleverly combines functional and naturopathic medicine with advanced dentistry. This book is biological dentistry at its absolute best."

**—Tim Gray**, biohacker; founder, Health Optimisation Summit

"A fascinating exploration of the fundamental connection between the health of your mouth, overall well-being, and your ability to perform on and off the field. An essential for anyone looking to reach their performance potential!"

**—Dr. Marc Bubbs**, ND, MSc, CISSN, CSCS, author of *Peak*

# It's All in Your MOUTH

**Biological Dentistry and the Surprising Impact of Oral Health on Whole Body Wellness**

## Dr. Dominik Nischwitz

Translated by Holly James

Chelsea Green Publishing
White River Junction, Vermont
London, UK

Editor: Brianne Goodspeed
Copy Editor: Laura Jorstad
Proofreader: Deborah Heimann
Indexer: Shana Milkie
Designer: Melissa Jacobson
Page Composition: Abrah Griggs

Printed in Canada.
First printing February 2020.
10 9 8 7 6 5 4 3 2 1    20 21 22 23

## Our Commitment to Green Publishing

Chelsea Green sees publishing as a tool for cultural change and ecological stewardship. We strive to align our book manufacturing practices with our editorial mission and to reduce the impact of our business enterprise in the environment. We print our books and catalogs on chlorine-free recycled paper, using vegetable-based inks whenever possible. This book may cost slightly more because it was printed on paper that contains recycled fiber, and we hope you'll agree that it's worth it. *It's All in Your Mouth* was printed on paper supplied by Marquis that is made of recycled materials and other controlled sources.

### Library of Congress Cataloging-in-Publication Data
Names: Nischwitz, Dominik, author.
Title: It's all in your mouth : biological dentistry and the surprising impact of oral health on whole body wellness / Dr. Dominik Nischwitz, Holly James ; translated by Holly James.
Other titles: In aller Munde English.
Description: White River Junction : Chelsea Green Publishing, [2020] | Includes bibliographical references and index.
Identifiers: LCCN 2019049737 (print) | LCCN 2019049738 (ebook) | ISBN 9781603589543 (paperback) | ISBN 9781603589550 (ebook)
Subjects: LCSH: Teeth—Care and hygiene. | Mouth—Care and hygiene. | Dental care.
Classification: LCC RK61 .N5613 2020 (print) | LCC RK61 (ebook) | DDC 617.6/01—dc23
LC record available at https://lccn.loc.gov/2019049737
LC ebook record available at https://lccn.loc.gov/2019049738

Chelsea Green Publishing
85 North Main Street, Suite 120
White River Junction, VT 05001

Somerset House
London, UK

www.chelseagreen.com

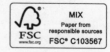

MIX
Paper from
responsible sources
FSC® C103567

*For my wife and soul mate, Steffi,*
*without whom I could never have done any of this.*

# CONTENTS

# PREFACE

When I was younger I wanted nothing more than to become a professional skater. I would use every free minute I had to practice, but each time I was about to reach the next stage of progression, I was held back by illness. For some reason my body was not as healthy or resistant as it should have been. Sometimes I would have a tonsil inflammation, sometimes a stubborn cold. I got shingles and glandular fever. My appendix became inflamed and had to be taken out. I had very bad skin, was always tired, and still found it difficult to sleep at night. I wanted to be fit, but instead I was constantly suffering from some ailment and had to undergo various courses of treatment. The medicines I took for my skin did help, but they had a negative effect on my liver. I was prescribed antibiotics again and again for my tonsil inflammation, until finally my doctor referred me to a surgeon to have them taken out.

This time my mother decided to take me to an alternative doctor, just to get a second opinion. After checking me over, he determined that I was allergic to dairy. At the time, I was eating and drinking copious amounts of milk and yogurt on a daily basis without ever wondering whether this could be having a negative effect on my health.

Up until that point I'd thought about illness in the same way most people do: You get sick, and you either take medication or have an operation, which you hope will make you better again, at least until the next bout of illness. We never did follow up on the referral to the surgeon, because once I stopped consuming dairy, the sore throats stopped. I didn't think too much about it, but somewhere in the back of my mind a lightbulb had been switched on: It became clear to me that there are ways to treat illness other than just taking medication all the time.

Despite this realization, I never did become a professional skater, and instead started my studies in dentistry. Sports were still important to me, but by this point it was weight training that had captured my imagination. When you want to build up muscles, you quickly learn that it takes more than just doing push-ups. It's also important to provide your body with all the right building blocks. I started learning about nutrition and taking note of the effects it had on me. At the time I was a student, and my life consisted of parties, minimal sleep, and bad food. Sometimes it felt like my body was ancient. Increasingly often, I also had spells of feeling low for no particular reason. So I decided to change a few things and was astounded at the effects that soon followed. There are certain foods that give us drive, and others that make us want to flop right back down on the sofa. I started opting more and more regularly for those that were doing me the most good. I started to wonder whether I could get my body into the condition that we are usually able to enjoy only in childhood, simply through diet and exercise. Is it possible to turn back the hands of time? I decided to work not only on building up my muscles, but also on getting my body into the healthiest condition possible.

My studies helped me to do precisely that. In my earlier school days, I found chemistry and physics so boring that I dropped them at the first opportunity. But now that I was studying them in direct relation to the human body, I found the subjects fascinating. What exactly is protein? How do carbohydrates work in the body? What is glycolysis? Which amino acids do we really need? Why are creatine and glutamine important? I had gone down various routes before finding the right thing for me: exercise and better nutrition. Soon I was fitter than I had ever been as a child or teenager.

My studies were coming to an end, but I wasn't particularly happy about it. I loved the practical and delicate work required in dentistry, but the rest I found oddly dissatisfying. There was something significant missing, but I couldn't put my finger on what. Then I took on an assistant's role in a dental practice specializing in surgery and implantology. The practice had been established many years prior, and my boss was one of the top experts in implantology. He was the perfect teacher and knew exactly how to get me motivated. The only problem was that he still used amalgam to fill dental cavities. Without really knowing why, I told my boss: "I'm sorry, but I can't do that."

At school we'd learned that amalgam is an easy material to work with that lasts for ages, isn't expensive, and kills bacteria. These fillings don't pose any kind of problem for most people, we were told; they just shouldn't be given to pregnant women or children. But I knew that my father, who is also a dentist, hadn't been using amalgam for twenty years because he didn't consider it to be healthy. If you make a bold statement like this as an assistant dentist, however, you need a stronger argument. As I didn't have one, I started to investigate that same day. I got increasingly carried away with what started off as a simple bit of research. I read studies and books; I attended seminars on the topic, learned about other dentists, doctors, and alternative practitioners; I watched videos and lectures and sat in on other dentists' procedures.

I'd only been looking for answers to a few questions, but what opened up before me was nothing less than a universe of information. I got to know dentists whose way of thinking was completely different from what I had learned during my studies. They didn't treat the mouth as an isolated body part. Instead they always took into account its relation to the rest of the body. It soon became clear to me that while some incredible technical feats are performed in dentistry, these can have devastating effects on our health in general.

Like all dentists, I had learned to concentrate on the mouth and teeth, but now I was beginning to learn about how the mouth and the rest of the organism are interwoven and only work as an inseparable whole. I realized that I knew a lot about how to fix teeth, but very little about what exactly causes dental problems in the first place—something that also had a lot to do with the rest of the body. Time and again I came across topics during this period that I had researched before because I personally found them interesting: nutrition, food, biochemistry, and the immune system. What seemed to be loose ends in my life suddenly came together. What had once interested me personally was now coming up again in my professional life. I discovered that, in my dentistry work, I wanted to focus on these connections. I wanted to be a dentist who doesn't just fix damage but tries to prevent it from happening in the first place. Finally, everything felt right.

Sometimes it takes only a few changes to make us feel better or get us back in good health. What I had achieved personally, I could now share with my patients. In fact, as a dentist I was in the perfect position to do so. I just had to add one or two pieces to the puzzle to complete it. I started to see my studies not as an end to my education but as the beginning. For five years I soaked up as much knowledge as possible. I learned about neural therapy, took the examination to become an alternative practitioner, and I learned about functional medicine, which treats the organism as a single, dynamic system in which everything is connected and works together, rather than dividing the body into different parts and specialist areas. I learned all about dental tools that can be used in the body without causing allergies or inflammation.

Today I have become the dentist that I always wanted to be. In 2015 my father and I opened the first Center for Biological Dentistry. This type of dentistry never treats the mouth as an isolated part of the body. Instead it focuses on the complex interactions that occur within the organism as a whole. I treat teeth, but every day I see how the whole body reacts to treatments when it is taken into account from the start of therapy. It is possible to live more healthily, to feel better, and to prevent diseases. My hope is that this book will enable me to share with others what I have known for years: Our mouths are the gateway to better overall health.

# Introduction

In 1957, a year before the World Cup was held in Sweden, Vicente Feola, coach of the Brazilian national soccer team, took some time to reflect like no other person before him had. Then he began to make detailed preparations for the upcoming contest. Of course he would need his most talented players and the very best training methods. But Feola wanted to think beyond that. He didn't want to overlook anything that might affect his players' performance, so he decided to take measures that had never before played a role in soccer training. Not only did he send his players to be checked over and looked after by a psychologist, but he also sent the entire team off to the dentist. And there was a lot of work to be done. Of the 470 teeth examined, 32 were diseased or inflamed and had to be taken out. When the Brazilians entered the competition a year later, they probably had the healthiest teeth of all participants.

Despite some particularly energy-sapping preliminaries, given how close the competition was, the Brazilians won the most confident and superior victory ever seen in the tournament.[1] From the outside Feola's methods seemed bizarre. Surely what soccer players need most are strapping calves, ball skills, and a lot of stamina? But today several studies have proven that the coach's intuition was spot-on: Good health and the best possible levels of fitness can only be attained if our mouths and teeth are all in good order.

For decades people thought that tooth decay and gum inflammation were the only types of disease it was possible to get in their mouths. But it's now been proven several times that cardiovascular diseases, diabetes, infertility, strokes, intestinal diseases, and many autoimmune diseases often begin in the mouth, or can be made worse by factors stemming from there. Diseased teeth, inflamed gums, and filling material rejected by the body do not only affect the mouth. Often their effects can be found in completely different places in the body in the form of knee problems, shoulder or back pain, or allergies that we can't quite seem to make sense of. Teeth that are diseased or poorly cared for deplete the body's energy and nutrients, which can initiate processes that trigger depression, affect our hormones and body chemistry, stimulate the immune system, and activate the stress axis twenty-four hours a day.

Today we know that the most chronic illnesses are not down to coincidence, bad luck, or bad genes. Instead they are the result of constant, silent inflammation in the body and the resulting chronic stress. This kind of inflammation often occurs in the mouth. It can be found hiding in the tips of inflamed tooth roots, gingival pockets, around implants, in dead teeth, or in the cavities that are left behind whenever a tooth has to be removed. Although research is constantly revealing new relationships between teeth and the body, this knowledge is far too infrequently used in practice. Doctors and dentists traditionally work in two separate spheres. A general practitioner will seldom look into the mouth, and a dentist's work is primarily technical.

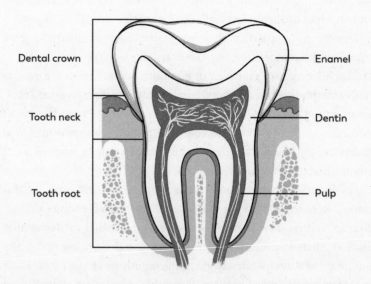

**Figure 0.1.** Hard on the outside, full of life on the inside. Underneath the visible enamel, each tooth is an organ in itself.

Our medical care system is structured such that we can't see the forest for the trees. What we desperately need is to look at the bigger picture. Up until now the mouth's role as the central organ that connects the two disciplines has been largely neglected, and with it the opportunity to understand the cause of many diseases as early as possible.

It's not only dentists who are taught to judge dental health according to whether the mouth's mechanical functions are in working order and whether the teeth are straight. Our teeth have to do a lot of work to break our food down into digestible pieces. But if we only see them as grinding machines that can be repaired when they break down, then we are doing them a huge injustice. This perspective also disregards what they really are and what role they play in our bodies. The visible part of our teeth is only a third of what is there. Sadly we never catch sight of the other exciting parts. And yet they ought to have attracted quite a bit of attention: At the core of each tooth lies, in the tiniest space, everything that constitutes an organ—pulsating blood vessels, lymph vessels, a nervous system, and an immune system. Like every other organ, our teeth are connected to the rest of the body via these systems. When the body is run down, our teeth suffer, too. If there is a problem with our teeth, it always has an effect on the rest of the body.

## A Paradigm Shift in Dentistry

Many of us make great efforts with our oral hygiene but end up feeling disappointed or even ashamed when our teeth become diseased despite regular brushing. For a long time the credo was: A clean tooth is a healthy tooth. Rows of products on supermarket shelves promise to provide the solution. We are offered a selection of interdental brushes, dental floss with added fluoride, antibacterial mouthwash . . . yet 95 percent of people suffer from tooth decay and 65 percent from gum disease. Many people soon become resigned to the idea that teeth simply aren't built to last. But some people's teeth don't even make it through the first four years of their lives. Our teeth are certainly made to last longer than that. Superficially fixing these patients' teeth in the same way we would give a car a new paint job isn't going to solve this problem. This is why it's so great that there are new ways of looking at the mouth that are changing the way we think about teeth and how they get diseased. Theories that have been considered valid for years are now coming under scrutiny and being corrected. A consensus has existed for a long time, but now a paradigm shift is taking place. We have learned to focus so much on fighting bad bacteria that we have lost sight of those that do us good and help promote good health. We've been concentrating so hard on cavities that we've forgotten about the mechanisms in place that make our teeth resilient and help them to constantly repair themselves. We've learned to see our teeth as inanimate objects, neglecting to ask ourselves whether they can even withstand the repair methods we have invented for them.

Biological dentistry brings together the overlooked factors, making connections and questioning traditions. It takes into account the sensitive biochemistry, physics, and biology of the body. As an organism, we have an enormous capacity to heal ourselves and are remarkably good at rejuvenating ourselves once the cause for any given disease is removed.

A new type of dentistry can help us do exactly that. Only a few of us are given the task of winning a World Cup. But most of us want to be able to stay healthy and active. For a long time people have been desperately seeking answers as to why they have become ill or just not as fit as they used to be. They want to know how they can take care of themselves—how they can get better and stay better. We should no longer overlook or deny the central role that our mouth has to play in answering these questions. Today we have so much more information available to us than the intuition that the coach of the Brazilian soccer team once had to rely on. We have new insights from the world of science that have enabled us to recognize connections in the body more clearly than ever before. We no longer have to content ourselves with snippets. We now have the whole picture.

Let the healing begin!

# Teeth and Microbiology

J ust over three hundred years ago, a young, restless Dutch man developed the strongest microscopic lens that had been ever been created in the world at the time. The man was in fact a draper called Antonie van Leeuwenhoek. But in his spare time, he was what would no doubt be described nowadays as a geek, something of an eccentric nerd. People in the textiles trade often used magnifying glasses for their work to judge the quality of fabrics. But van Leeuwenhoek also loved to use them to explore his environment. He studied beetles' legs, flies' probosces, bees' eyes, and the structure of leaves with endless fascination. He discovered that another, multifaceted world existed beyond the one we can perceive with the naked eye. This world is perceptible to us if only we could zoom in close enough. So he learned how to cut lenses and worked independently to design and make increasingly effective models. He had already worked on over 550 lenses when he finally built a microscope that could magnify objects to 275 times their size.

With this mega magnifying device, he discovered that blood was not just a viscous red liquid, but was in fact made up of individual, tightly packed red blood cells. By the same means, van Leeuwenhoek debunked the existing conception of the spontaneous creation of species when he discovered that semen was teeming with millions of minuscule sperm. Having realized that everything that seemed so familiar at first glance was in fact full of unknown secrets revealed only upon closer inspection, he scratched off some of the white film that, as we all know, builds up after a few hours of not brushing our teeth, and examined it under his microscope. It turned out that this film, too, contained something very surprising, something quite extraordinary: It was teeming with living organisms. Some were small and round, others rather long; some simply sat immobile, while some wriggled around blithely. Van Leeuwenhoek could not make head nor tail of these organisms, so he simply named them *dierkens*, or little animals. He had no idea that in the blink of an eye, he had discovered an entire species: microorganisms. Single-celled organisms were completely unheard of up until this point, which is why van Leeuwenhoek had trouble trying to convince anyone of their existence for a very a long time. He even faced serious questioning as a result of his observations. Hundreds of years of technical advances later, their existence is no longer doubted by anyone, but we still haven't quite come to grips with these extraordinary cohabitants of the human body.

What scientists are sure of is that microorganisms such as bacteria, fungi, and viruses are some of the toughest, most persistent creatures in the entire world. We can trace their existence back to the Big Bang, some 13.8 billion years ago. Microorganisms even had the earth to themselves for three billion years, until other forms of life came to join them. They simply adjusted to living with every new living being that appeared, and to this day they can settle on just about any material. They live on plants, hang out on animals, and can be found in all types of soil, sediment, and rock. They can live a comfortable existence on glacial ice, hot springs, or radioactive deserts.

Some have even left earth on spacecraft. But microorganisms don't just sit there doing nothing; they play an active role in shaping the world and everything in it. There are clear traces of them in all habitats on earth. And one of those habitats happens to be human beings.

## Oral Microbia: The Discovery of a New World

Microorganisms like our bodies so much that no sooner is a new human born than they begin to pounce. The first single-celled organisms settle on the body as we are being pushed out of the birth canal. In the womb a baby is more or less sterile, but as soon as it opens its mouth for the very first time to cry, the first organisms move in and start to make themselves at home. And these first settlers don't get to keep the place to themselves for long. There are two pretty strong human instincts that make sure of this throughout the rest of our lives:

1. We get hungry.
2. We want to find out what kind of a world we live in.

During the first week of our lives, our eyes are virtually blind, and we're not even aware of the fact that we've got hands yet. But we do have a mouth. Our entire existence revolves around the oral cavity: We are essentially nothing but a hungry, curious mouth. We use it not only to eat but also as our most important organ for experiencing the world around us. It is no accident that it is the organ most closely linked to the brain, to which it is connected via the strongest nerve in our body—the trigeminal nerve—in the most direct way possible. Until around three years of age, we slobber our way around the world, because we can understand the nature of objects and surfaces much more precisely with our mouths than with our hands, which only begin to develop their sense of touch much later on. While we are

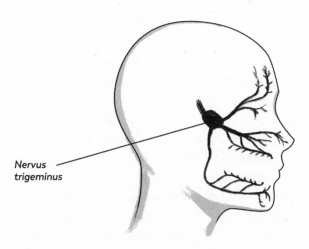

Nervus
trigeminus

**Figure 1.1.** Our teeth are directly connected to the brain via the strongest nerve in our body, the *nervus trigeminus*, or trigeminal nerve.

## A Little Glossary of Our Invisible Cohabitants

We often think of bacteria in black-and-white terms, as either good or bad. But in reality they each have quite a wide variety of characteristics—almost as many as humans. Some are more self-sufficient than others, some are sensitive, some are very agile, and others lethargic.

Microbiologists' categorization of these characteristics, of course, is a little more complex. They separate the mini inhabitants of our mouths into four main groups: commensal, symbiotic, pathogenic, and opportunistic microorganisms, which can usually live alongside one another in symbiosis, despite their differences.

Commensal bacteria can be classified as neither good nor bad. They are simply there to dine alongside their hosts—humans—which is neither an advantage nor a disadvantage to us.

hard at work filling our heads with information about our surroundings in this way, our mouths simultaneously fill up with more and more new inhabitants.

There are a lot of microorganisms coming and going in our mouths during those first few years. Depending on the conditions in our mouths at any given time, different microorganisms feel particularly at home in their environment. When a child is being weaned from breastfeeding, for example, certain microorganisms pack their bags and disappear along with their favorite means of subsistence: maternal milk. At the same time, others that prefer to feed on something a little more substantial begin to move in along with milk replacements. Others still will only drop by when our first teeth start to come through; these organisms prefer to make their homes where these

This is not the case with symbiotic bacteria: They stick with their hosts through thick and thin. The products of their metabolism are good both for us and for the microbial community as a whole.

Certain bacteria in the commensal category are also described as opportunistic, because this is exactly how they behave: Most of the time they are completely harmless, unless they have the opportunity to grow and band together with kindred spirits. Once they reach a certain number, they trigger diseases, making them pathogenic.

In a balanced system, they simply live alongside other microorganisms and are completely harmless. This group includes the notorious streptococcus, which we are particularly afraid of.

We only notice their presence in our bodies when we are ill, but they can in fact be part of a completely healthy flora. A strep smear, which parents often insist on having when their children have a fever, is therefore generally of little use.

hard substances begin to appear. From the moment we start to get our milk teeth to the arrival of our permanent teeth, the ecological conditions in our mouths change several times, as does the composition of the microbial community. Once we reach adulthood, each of us has acquired our own typical composition that is unique to us. Microbiologists also describe these microbes as "resident microflora" because they usually stay relatively stable—under favorable conditions—and live in balance with a wide variety of cohabitants. Often microbes that are not able to thrive in this environment also show up, but as long as the ecosystem is not disturbed they have a hard time settling down and soon disappear again.

Generally we think good oral health requires a mouth that is "clean" or low in bacteria. In reality our mouths are only healthy when they are teeming with thriving microorganisms. Stability and balance among the different types of microorganisms are more important than sterility. Researchers continue to count them, but so far they have been able to find around seven hundred different species of microbe, which all belong to a regular oral flora and even carry out several useful tasks. Promises from mouthwash companies to provide us with the best dental care with their antibacterial products are therefore questionable. These ads are based on relatively old ways of thinking.

While van Leeuwenhoek described bacteria rather neutrally—if not lovingly—as little animals, they developed quite a bad image later on. Since scientists and doctors discovered that they were responsible for infections, bacteria have come under general suspicion of causing illnesses. For decades we have thought of them as lurking parasites that must be fought against. We clean our houses with disinfectant household cleaning substances, wash ourselves with antimicrobial soaps, and eat animals that have been fed with antibiotics. Luckily we are now starting to look at microorganisms in a slightly different way. When van Leeuwenhoek looked though a very strong microscope over three hundred years ago, he discovered living beings that were able to live closely alongside us. The powerful magnifying glasses that we have access to today enable us to see much more. We are now able to get to know these microorganisms better, and often find them to be thoroughly pleasant little creatures.

## Tiny Cells with a Big Impact

Let's start by taking a trip into the world of economics. When companies grow and are no longer able or willing to do everything by themselves, they employ a strategy known as outsourcing. This simply means they entrust certain areas of responsibility to a subsidiary company. These companies can often provide services much more efficiently, giving the parent company more time for attending to core business. Of course, this is often a highly effective way for these companies to save money, as other workers can potentially carry out this work at a cheaper rate than company employees.

It is not entirely clear why our bodies outsource certain tasks, but we are certain that they make full use of this strategy. The body outsources things that we would assume belong to its core activities, such as metabolism. Metabolism, or digestion, refers to the process that occurs when our body converts a cheese sandwich into energy, nutrients, and hundreds of other little building blocks that are perfectly adapted to maintain all the different parts of the body and keep it strong.

Food undergoes many—mostly chemical—processes that transform it from one substance into another before taking on the most suitable form for the body's purposes.

We assume, for example, that we absorb vitamins by eating fruit. But our bodies absorb vitamin K thanks to certain bacteria that

## Man or Microbe?

If we were to count every single cell in our body, we would find around thirty billion in the average human being. If we add the cells of all the microorganisms living in and on our bodies, the figure increases significantly to thirty-nine billion. All in all we can safely say that we are more human than microbe. Certain medical researchers recommend that we no longer focus exclusively on humans, but consider ourselves as the sum of all our organisms, because we can only function with them. Some go as far as to say that bacteria do not only populate humans, but that they *are* us. Together with our microorganisms, humans form superorganisms known as holobionts. Only when we learn to understand the body as a whole can we truly understand how it works and consequently, how it becomes ill and can recover. The most important thing to remember is that most illnesses are caused by a disruption to the relationship between humans and microbes.

produce it for us in the form we need. Our body then says a friendly "thanks!" before passing it on to the liver, which can use it to build clotting factors that stop bleeding when we injure ourselves.

Other bacteria produce, for example, the neurotransmitter serotonin—much more even than what is produced by our brains, which was assumed to be the main source of serotonin for a long time.[1] Serotonin ensures that our moods remain stable and helps us to feel less anxious. Incidentally, the gut is another central location for other neurotransmitters: A total of 95 percent of neurotransmitters are cultivated there. Bodies and microorganisms are therefore busy working together at all times.

When bacteria break down fiber, for example, short-chain fatty acids are produced. This is something that so-called microglia are very happy about. Microglia police the immune system, keeping germs and dead nerve cells out of our brains to keep them healthy. So eating a lot of fiber is therefore good not only for our digestive systems, but also for our heads. Overall, roughly 30 percent of all metabolic products in our blood are of microbial origin. They strengthen our immune systems, produce anti-inflammatory substances, and regulate our digestive systems. Although people used to think that bacteria were putting our health at risk, more and more people are coming to the conclusion that it's actually the other way around: Without bacteria, our health is at risk.

## Back-to-Front Biology: The Somewhat Late Discovery of the Mouth

Despite the fact that the mouth is quite clearly the entrance to our gastrointestinal tract, scientists have taken a back-to-front approach to studying the digestive system, so to speak. Many of the fascinating findings about our coexistence with bacteria have many come from examinations of the intestine. No other organ has received quite so much attention in recent years. In 2001 seventy-nine studies were carried out on the subject. This number rose to over seven thousand in 2016.[2] And no wonder: It's the perfect place for studying the symbiosis of man and microbe. Nowhere else in the human body is the number and variety of microorganisms as great as in the intestine. Nowhere else in the human body do they take on as many tasks. Gradually, however, scientists are starting to direct their gazes upward: specifically, to the mouth and its impact on the intestine.

Anatomically, the mouth and the gastrointestinal tract are hardly distinguishable. Our mouths are not isolated units that simply stop after the uvula. In fact, the border between the mouth and intestine only exists in anatomy books. In real life they make up an inseparable unit. Every strain of bacteria in our intestine has made its way there via our mouths, and we now know that the microbial populations of oral and intestinal flora remain strongly connected throughout our lives. This is due in no small part to the fact that our saliva contains up to 109 microorganisms per milliliter, which make their way into the intestine each time we swallow. That's one to three grams of bacteria per day.[3]

The close connection between the mouth and intestine has many advantages for humans. Visibility is one of them. While it's quite difficult to look at our intestines without a technical device to find out what's going on in there, it's quite easy to look inside our mouth. We simply have to open it and have a look. Sometimes it's not even necessary to do that. It's possible to tell when someone has a health problem with their mouth simply by smelling it. Bad breath is almost always an indication of an imbalance in the microbial community. An imbalance in the oral flora might smell acrid, sour, sulfurous, or—in the case of severe inflammation—like a festering open wound.

An entrance hall will usually tell you what to expect to find in the rest of the building. Our mouths work in the same way. If there is an unfavorable bacterial climate here because our gums or the tooth root are chronically inflamed or because bad tooth fillings are constantly releasing toxic substances, then this problem does not stop somewhere beyond the tonsils. Inflamed oral mucosa always continue farther down into the intestine. If the ecology in the mouth becomes imbalanced, this usually affects our remaining gastrointestinal apparatus as well. And what you see in the mouth usually continues into the gut. Recently researchers discovered that inflammatory bowel diseases such as Crohn's or ulcerative colitis may originate in oral microbia. Scientists have found increased numbers of bacteria types that are usually found in the mouth in the intestinal microbia of people with diseases. It would appear that a particular genus of these bacteria can cause intestinal inflammation in people with a predisposition (a susceptibility) to particular diseases when they are swallowed with saliva.[4]

For some time now the importance of the considerable microbial community in our mouths has become the focus of research. But there's always room for us to gain a better understanding of what exactly is going on in there.

## Life in the Mouth: Heaven or Hell?

If you ask a person to imagine an ideal world, they will probably talk about world peace and an abundance of food for everyone. Ask a dentist what a perfect mouth looks like, and they'll tell you it's one in which there is a positive symbiosis between hosts and microbes. In reality these two visions are not worlds apart: Many different beings living alongside one another, with enough provisions for everyone. The host—that is, the human—is always a winner in this ideal situation. When microbes are able to coexist in our mouths, none of the bacteria living there harm us. The community works diligently to keep our teeth and gums healthy. For microorganisms, however, such a place can be heaven and hell at the same time.

One the one hand the mouth is an attractive place for microbes to live. It is always warm and moist—conditions that bacteria love more than anything. There are lots of different nooks and surfaces that make excellent hideouts, and every time the front door opens, the food supplies are replenished. On the other hand life can be hellish in the mouth, which can also be a very inhospitable place. There's constant chewing, speaking, breathing, brushing, and rinsing going on. If bacteria want to set up camp here, they have to learn one thing above all: how to hold on. But bacteria wouldn't have been able to survive for almost four billion years on earth if they didn't have a few tricks up their sleeves. And one of their most spectacular ones is known as the biofilm.

## Biofilm: Clinging On for Dear Life

Microorganisms are minuscule and are each made up exclusively of a single cell. But there is one significant characteristic that makes them uncannily like humans: They don't like to live alone. When a group of humans comes together, we call this a community. When bacteria join together, scientists call this a biofilm. This might sound a like some kind of quality label, but it actually refers to the complex matrix that is created when millions of microorganisms decide to settle together on a surface to create a new living environment with the optimal conditions for themselves. In the past dentists would often warn patients about plaque, by which they meant the white, sticky layer that builds up on our teeth whenever we forget to brush them. Plaque was something we were all told to avoid. But now plaque is a thing of the past. Today we look at this layer a little differently. Long before we can see or feel plaque, bacteria have already joined together to form a complex community: biofilm. We only speak of plaque once the biofilm has reached a certain thickness. So even when we have the feeling that our teeth are clean, because they feel nice and smooth when we run our tongues over them, there are already quite a few extraordinary things happening on them. The microscopically small complexes that begin to emerge could rival the Mayan cities of Guatemala.

Forming a biofilm to stay strong is not something microbes have come up with specifically for our mouths. They have been doing it for millions of years wherever they end up. Biofilms can also be found, for example, as the slippery deposits on the underside of a boat or as the layer that attaches itself to the pole of a jetty. In our bodies biofilms can also be found in places other than the mouth, where they are not always as harmless. We now know, for example, that they are involved in the formation of deposits in blood vessels, known as atherosclerosis or calcium deposits. This type of plaque is often composed of films of bacteria from the mouth, which demonstrates one of the ways in which the mouth is closely linked to the heart.[5] A bacterial community can usually adhere to any surface thanks to biofilm. But in the mouth, this is particularly tricky. The structure

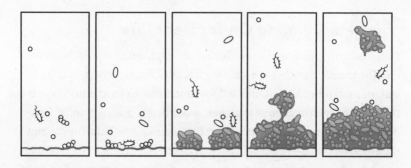

**Figure 1.2.** Biofilm microorganisms form complex structures on our teeth after just a short amount of time.

of teeth means that just about everything slips off them. To attach something to them is like trying to nail jelly to a wall. Luckily for bacteria, there's something quite special on hand that acts a little bit like an anti-slip mat . . .

## The Pellicle: A Magic Shield for Our Teeth

What can you expect to find in the average mouth? To start with, there should be thirty-two teeth. Then of course you've got the gums and the tongue. Then there is the pellicle. If you've never heard of it before, don't worry. Even scientists overlooked the pellicle for a very long time. Yet we can clearly feel it when we run our tongue over our teeth. Most of us think that it's just saliva coating our teeth and making them so wonderfully smooth. It's true that saliva has something to do with this smoothness, but perhaps not in the way we would expect. Our teeth are not just moistened by saliva; in fact they are permanently coated in a delicate, transparent net. Scientists have named this coating the pellicle. This film is broken several times a day, for example when we brush our teeth, or as a result of abrasion when we eat something hard, like a carrot. It's not a problem, however, because the pellicle can re-form in the blink of an eye, over and over again.

The process really is magical. No sooner have we brushed our teeth than this netlike film begins to re-form, until it completely covers our teeth again. Those who have studied the pellicle extensively have come to the conclusion that it is more than just a by-product that forms in the mouth; it is in fact an entity, a unit in itself, just like the tongue or teeth. We can also picture the pellicle as a kind of stationary saliva. While saliva flows around our teeth, the pellicle has the properties of a solid and sticks to our teeth. This is why it's also described as autochthonous. That might sound a little technical, but the discovery of an autochthonous texture for teeth is like a dream come true for scientists: A substance that is able to protect the teeth as well and as discreetly as the pellicle could be used, for example, to help to protect teeth from tooth decay. To this day all attempts to re-create the pellicle have failed. Any material applied to the teeth is inevitably washed away soon after. The pellicle therefore continues to be studied intensively.

That said, some of the pellicle's secrets have already been revealed. In the beginning each pellicle is made up of proteins that come from food. These start to settle just seconds after we finish brushing our teeth. We could even say that our teeth attract the pellicle to them. This is because the calcium ions in enamel are positively charged and attract the protein building blocks like magnets. As soon as they settle, the process looks something like Tetris. Gradually, other building blocks such as biomolecules, macromolecules, mucins, enzymes, and antibacterial agents like lysozyme, cystatins, and histatins are deposited on the teeth. You don't need to know all of these substances; it's probably enough just to know that they are all quite good for our teeth. After thirty to ninety minutes, the pellicle has reached its maximum thickness. It may only be visible on a nanoscopic scale, but that's enough for it to perform some very important functions.

Thanks to the pellicle our teeth glide past one another as we chew without grinding one another down. This protection is very important because our teeth are exposed to grinding through chewing up to fifteen thousand times per day, often with a bite force of several pounds. Without any form of lubricant, they would quickly wear down.

At the same time, our teeth are protected from poisons, carcinogens, mechanical damage, and acids by this delicate coating.

## A Fat Lot of Good

We can actively help the pellicle do its job by eating the right types of food. Studies have shown that the more lipids—fats—our foods contain, the better and stronger the pellicle becomes. Even rinsing with olive oil, aloe vera, or coconut oil seems to have a positive effect on the fat content of the pellicle. Those who swear by oil pulling, an alternative medicine practice that involves rinsing with oil, might just be onto something.

But the pellicle is never left in peace for long. Around half an hour after it reaches maximum thickness, the first bacteria begin to settle. Some of them do this by association—biologists' term for the relatively loose connection between bacteria and surfaces. These pioneers use their physical strength to grasp onto the pellicle, where they get to kick back for a while. Subsequent arrivals are a little more forceful and claw themselves onto special surface molecules. The pellicle is electrostatically charged to prevent precisely that from happening. But microorganisms are cunning creatures. Some of them can simply form protons and cations to neutralize the electrostatic charge on the pellicle. Others manage to get around the barrier by other means: They don't cling to the surface of the teeth at all, instead grabbing onto the first settlers.

In other words, they grab onto other microorganisms that were already there before them. It's hard to say whether the first settlers give their lives up for the greater good like martyrs or whether they are simply crushed by their successors. In any case, many of the pioneer bacteria die shortly after the others arrive. The bacteria bringing up the rear then make short work of creating what are known as micro-colonies. The microbes organize themselves, split up tasks, and create transport routes for their degradation products. They communicate well with one another to ensure that each task is carried out swiftly in a controlled way.

Believe it or not, microorganisms really do communicate with one another. In fact, they have more and better ways of doing so than we humans do. They communicate via physical contact by exchanging metabolic products or passing signaling molecules to one another. If an organism from another species needs a certain piece of information urgently, it's not a problem. There's no such thing as language barriers in their world. Viruses can happily chat with bacteria, who in turn natter away with fungi. In our world this would be like everyone

## We Need to Talk . . .

For decades, we have had only one weapon to fight against infections: antibiotics. There are various categories, but generally speaking they are all used to break down the cell walls of bacteria or to intervene in metabolic processes to prevent them from spreading any further. Unfortunately, this not only affects the organisms causing the problem; it also affects many innocent bystanders that normally only do good. Researchers are therefore looking for new treatment methods. There are currently attempts under way to manufacture antibiotics that don't simply eliminate bacteria, but instead make them communicate differently with one another. This is because bacteria usually only make us sick when the number of them in our bodies has exceeded a critical point. They are able to do this, above all, as a result of effective organization and communication. Thanks to cellular communication, also known as quorum sensing, bacteria are able to tell one another how many of them are present in their immediate environment and how they can get connected. The new generation of antibiotics works by disrupting the communication between biomolecules in a targeted way.[6]

on earth being able to communicate not only with one another, but also with elephants, llamas, and even zebra finches, all using the same language. Some people dream of a world in which everyone can speak Esperanto. Microorganisms have been communicating in a single language since time immemorial.

Clearly there's a lot more to microbes than meets the eye. We simply don't know enough about them yet. The advantages of a biofilm, on the other hand, are obvious. Organisms are stronger and more effective together than they are alone. They can withstand external attacks and food shortages. Within a biofilm, they even have the most powerful weapon known to humankind: antibiotics.

At a certain point bacteria begin to form extracellular polysaccharides within the biofilm. In other words, they produce a sort of coating they can safely encase themselves in. It's only when too many of the wrong types of bacteria entrench themselves in this way and become unmanageable that they become harmful to humans. The mouth has a secret weapon, however, that can help it to prevent this from happening under the right conditions. What is this all-purpose weapon? Saliva.

## Saliva: Underrated Miracle Water

Saliva is something we often find a little disgusting when it's not in its rightful place: the mouth. But saliva is truly a miracle weapon. Most people are surprised to find out that we produce up to a quart and a half of saliva a day. Saliva becomes really fascinating, however, when we take a closer look at what it carries and what different tasks it performs simultaneously. Ninety-five percent of saliva is exactly what it looks like: water. But the remaining 5 percent is so complex that to this day, researchers haven't managed to fully identify all of its contents. So far over two thousand elements have been identified, but at the moment we only know the exact functions of the most important ones. What we do know is that saliva provides a true cocktail of nutrients. It contains several minerals including calcium, magnesium, sodium, potassium, iron, and copper. The main reason saliva contains these nutrients is to supply our teeth with them.

## Fluoride: The Best Means of Fighting Tooth Decay?

Fluoride is considered an essential part of dental care. Almost all toothpaste contains it, and it is also used in high doses for most professional prophylaxis procedures (but not in holistic dentistry). The fact that the spread of tooth decay has declined in the last few years is therefore often linked to the widespread use of fluoride. Some states in the United States add it to the water. In Germany, however, no fluoride is added to drinking water—and yet rates of tooth decay have dropped. Fluoride is able to store and lock calcium and other minerals in tooth enamel, which sounds like a wonderful, helpful attribute. But whenever something has a positive effect on the body, a side effect is usually not far behind. There are endless studies linking fluoride to chromosomal changes, bone cancer, and impairments to intelligence, while as many other studies still declared it innocent of such allegations. In any case, it has never been fully acquitted; the consensus is that fluoride is toxic above certain thresholds. Fluoride advocates argue that this limit cannot be exceeded through toothpaste use alone. The concept of holistic dentistry, however, is based on avoiding overburdening the body with artificial substances as far as possible. If we eat well and get all the nutrients we need, there is no need for additional fluoride. Saliva's job is to store minerals in teeth. That is its natural function, and it does not require extra fluoride to get the job done. Milk teeth are the exception to this rule; see "Dental Care for Children" on page 160 for more information on fluoride.

To understand how this works, it's worth getting to know the uppermost layer of our teeth: tooth enamel. Ninety-eight percent of tooth enamel is composed of minerals such as calcium, phosphorus, magnesium, and fluoride, which is what makes it so hard. Chemists would describe this kind of substance as inorganic, which means it is not a living substance. This doesn't mean that nothing is going on in tooth enamel, however. Even if we don't notice it when we look in the mirror, there are highly dynamic processes constantly taking place on our teeth. Tooth enamel might be the strongest tissue in the human body, but it begins to dissolve as soon as the pH values in its environment drops—in other words, becomes acidic.

Given that we now eat many foods that lower the pH in our mouths, elements such as calcium and phosphorus are continuously released from tooth enamel as we eat and chew.

In a way each of us has a very mild form of tooth decay during the course of the day. But it isn't a problem if our teeth have the opportunity to recharge the lost substances often enough and for long enough. This process is known as remineralization. This is a crucial mechanism for the health of our teeth, and saliva provides the perfect assistance. Not only does it supply our teeth with the nutrients they require, it also provides buffer substances like phosphate and bicarbonate, which they use to neutralize acidity and produce a base pH value that enables remineralization to happen in the first place. In an acidic environment, the process is simply stopped.

While its main purpose in the past was fighting plaque, today saliva is becoming increasingly important in the prevention of tooth decay and gum disease. In dental laboratories there is so much focus on saliva that it now has its own parameters. We study how fast cars travel in miles per hour, storms in wind speed. When scientists want to find out the average amount of saliva produced in the human mouth, the parameter is known as clearance rate. The reason why salivation rate is significant is that there isn't always enough saliva in the mouth. Many people's rate is sometimes low, while others barely salivate at all. A low clearance rate leads to a more significant and persistent drop in the pH of the saliva—and therefore in the biofilm—which has a detrimental effect on the teeth. However, there are certain circumstances that permanently lower pH levels because they take place directly in the mouth. Dental materials such as amalgam (used for fillings) and other metals can create a more acidic pH level. The

## More Fluids, Less Decay

We've all experienced dry mouth when we're nervous or have to give a speech in public. This is because these situations equal stress. Under stress our bodies slow down the production of all digestive functions, and this includes saliva. Under chronic stress this can become a permanent condition. The lower the salivation rate in our mouths, the higher the risks of tooth decay. Dry mouth is a very common phenomenon. Around a quarter of Germans suffer from it.[7]

In old age saliva production rates tend to decline. According to one study almost 40 percent of patients over the age of sixty suffer from dry mouth, which is also related to systemic diseases such as diabetes. Dry mouth is also a common side effect of over four hundred medicines, including those used to treat hay fever, high blood pressure, depression, and epileptic seizures. As we attempt to control an illness with medication on the one hand, we may be putting ourselves at risk of tooth decay on the other. Salivary deficiency can also simply arise as a result of not drinking enough. Even if total body fluid drops by only 3 percent, salivary production reduces significantly. Sometimes simply drinking more and chewing a sugar-free chewing gum can help the salivary glands jump back into action again.

higher the salivation rate, the higher the proportion of calcium, inorganic phosphates, and bicarbonates, which play an important role in preventing tooth decay. The higher the salivation rate, the stronger the concentration of these nutrients.

The impact of saliva and the pH value in the mouth, however, is even more far reaching. Not only does it provide the teeth with nutrients, it also has a great impact on the microbe community. A permanently low pH value significantly reduces the diversity of microorganisms compared with a higher value, and under certain circumstances creates favorable circumstances for pathogenic bacteria.

Antibacterial substances are not only produced by the pharmaceutical industry; our mouths are capable of producing them independently. We even subconsciously use these substances—for example, when we cut a finger our reflex is to put the injured finger into our mouth. And this can have quite a significant effect. Our saliva contains a peptide called histatin, which kills pathogenic germs, promotes quicker healing of wounds, and stops blood from flowing.

Saliva also contains a significant proportion of immunoglobulins. These substances attack pathogenic microorganisms directly or limit their growth to ensure that they do not take over the mouth.

Mucins help with this process, too. These are fluids that give saliva its typical, slightly slimy consistency. Mucins are truly multi-talented, because they work simultaneously in several different ways: They prevent certain pathogenic bacteria from collecting and settling in one place. They do not inhibit these bacteria; rather, they make them

## Tough Foods Make You Tougher

You might have heard it said that food well chewed is easier to digest. But it's also worth knowing that properly chewing our food can help to protect us from infections. Researchers recently discovered this when they took a closer look at what are known as Th17 cells in our mouths. These cells are part of the immune system and can ward off bacteria that are harmful to our health, while leaving friendly bacteria in peace. Th17 cells form in the mouth; the more we chew, the more cells are produced. Eating foods with a tougher consistency, or simply chewing well, ensures a better immune defense in the mouth.[8]

more mobile. When mucins are present, microbes behave as though they are on Ecstasy. They become so fidgety that settling down is the last thing on their minds. Mucins also make it difficult for these bad bacteria to communicate with one another; then they collect them up in one place and transport them away. Researchers have also noted that certain streptococcus varieties multiply quickly in the absence of saliva, while their growth remains moderate within it. Saliva really does have the power to keep certain bacteria in check and therefore ensure that a balance is established in the bacteria community.[9]

## Microbial Homeostasis: Oral Health in the Balance

Our mouths have all sorts of secret weapons for protecting our teeth from harmful bacteria, acidity, mechanical damage, and all other negative influences. They are constantly being rinsed, food particles washed away, the pH value neutralized, plaque rubbed off, and our teeth tirelessly remineralized when the enamel loses important substances. All of these measures ensure a condition that biologists and dentists call microbial homeostasis. This means that bacteria are abundant in our mouths, but there is a stable and balanced relationship among them. In this harmonious setting the microbial community is doing us a lot of good and is working to keep our mouths and the rest of the body healthy.

However, homeostasis is a condition that is not usually long lasting; it constantly needs to be reestablished. Homoeostasis can be imagined as a kind of punching bag. Although it repeatedly has to withstand strong blows, the bag is always able to spring back to a central position. Each time the harmony in the mouth is compromised, there are many self-regulating mechanisms in place to restore the original balance immediately. Despite this, homeostasis can sometimes break down. Any form of disease in the mouth is precisely that: a lasting imbalance between the mini inhabitants there. This happens when the blows are too strong and we are no longer able to bounce back to the center. If the balance in the mouth is disrupted for any length of time, bacteria that cause diseases gain the upper hand.

A punching bag is designed to be able to withstand a high number of blows, but our bodies are not. At least, they aren't designed for the strain they have to undergo nowadays. When a system was designed to keep our mouths healthy, clearly nobody had thought of lollipops, orange soda, cigarette smoke, alcohol, or gold and amalgam fillings. Nor did anyone envision the antibiotic treatments or constant stress that lower our defenses and affect our salivation levels. Our mouths can withstand a lot, but in the world we live in, we overwhelm their protective mechanisms far too often. The symbiosis in which we used to live then changes. It becomes a dysbiosis, which is the opposite. In a dysbiosis the dental diseases that wreak the most havoc with our mouths are allowed to thrive: tooth decay and gum disease.

## Tooth Decay: A New Way of Thinking About an Old Disease

The model according to which tooth decay operates seemed so easy that it could easily be made into a children's story: Two bacteria live together in the same tooth, and because the person in question rarely brushes their teeth, the bacteria get stronger and decide to spread to other teeth and even start using pickaxes to make some changes to the place. Only once the owner goes to the dentist to remove the bacteria's new structures and start to brush their teeth regularly do the two villains pull up stakes and go looking for another child for whom dental hygiene isn't a big priority.

There are certain diseases that are highly complicated and puzzling, but tooth decay seems quite simple. Everyone learns about how it develops and how to avoid it. And yet: Tooth decay is the world's most common disease. Ninety-five percent of adults find a cavity in one or more teeth over the course of their lifetime. Either seven billion people are doing something wrong, despite the guidelines, or there's more to the development of tooth decay than we once thought.

For centuries a "worm" was said to be responsible for tooth decay. Holes in fruits and vegetables do not look dissimilar to those in teeth, and anyone who has experienced toothache would agree that they have experienced a sensation of gnawing. But a new age brought with it new theories. These were initially presented by Wiloughby William Miller, a student of microbiologist Robert Koch. In 1890 Miller discovered that bacteria in the oral flora convert carbohydrates into acids, and that these acids lead to the decalcification of teeth.

Bacteria then settle in the resulting lesions and continue to destroy the tooth structure. To this day Miller is considered a pioneer in dentistry and dental hygiene, but the foundation of our modern understanding of tooth decay was established decades later thanks to a couple of hamsters. That's right, hamsters.

Well, they weren't just any hamsters; they were gnotobiotic hamsters. Gnotobiotic animals are often used in medical research. They are bred and raised in such a way that they remain virtually free of germs. Observations showed that even if they were fed large quantities of sucrose, they never developed tooth decay. But if they were put in a cage together with other hamsters that did have tooth decay, or ate the feces of these hamsters, they, too, soon began to develop cavities. The same thing happened when researchers transferred isolated bacteria from hamsters with tooth decay to healthy rodents. But when this group was treated with antibiotics, they remained cavity-free. Suddenly everything became clear. Tooth decay was a contagious disease. A children's book was created with the characters Karius and Bactus to explain this phenomenon, but in medicine it is referred to as the specific plaque hypothesis. The focus was now on *Streptococcus mutans*, and a few other types of lactobacillus, all of which are considered to be acidogenic and acidophilic (acid forming and acid loving).

In the field of oral hygiene, a similar approach was adopted to the one used in infectiology: To avoid getting cavities, we must avoid the transmission of acidic bacteria, preventing its spread or, ideally, eliminating it completely. It even got to the point that parents were urged not to let their children come into contact with certain things: Don't suck a baby's pacifier when it falls on the floor, don't eat from the same spoon, and ideally, don't even kiss your children to avoid bacteria that cause tooth decay to be transmitted via saliva.

What's more, oral hygiene practices were primarily based on the chemical or mechanical removal of dental plaque. These were followed by attempts to use antibiotics in toothpaste, as well as vaccines against

## A Losing Battle

For a long time people were convinced that they could control bacteria. All it took was to identify, categorize, and finally fight them, whenever we wanted to overcome disease. But the complexity of these creatures has thrown a spanner in the works. The better our measuring instruments become, the more varieties of bacteria we discover. The abundance is sometimes a shock for scientists. We know that there are more than seven hundred types in a healthy mouth. If we look at oral flora with high-throughput technology, the number increases to nineteen hundred. To kill every single type of bacteria that lives in the biofilm, we would need antibiotics at 300x concentration. But humans could never survive a dose of this strength.[10]

tooth decay.[11] This was the age of the dentist who would issue friendly but stern warnings about brushing teeth twice a day or after each meal. The credo was "clean teeth are healthy teeth," and controlling tooth decay focused on eliminating the bacteria that people believed were the culprits.

The hamster experiments were followed by numerous further investigations and cross-sectional studies on humans. But instead of providing clarity and confirmation, they revealed inconsistencies that did not fit prior assumptions:

1. Several studies showed that children with good oral hygiene were less likely to develop tooth decay than children who brushed less regularly. That said, the differences in each case were negligible.[12]

2. Some people brush regularly, rinse and floss until their mouths are as clean as operating theaters, yet they still suffer from tooth decay.

3. It has been discovered that some people with tooth decay do not
   have any trace of *Streptococcus mutans* on their teeth whatsoever.
4. Certain people in developing countries, on the other hand, have
   high concentrations of *Streptococcus mutans* on their teeth, but
   do not have a particularly high proportion of tooth decay.[13]

The specific plaque theory developed in the past was now being
questioned. Today researchers have come to the conclusion that
*Streptococcus mutans* is not a pathogen per se—which is to say it
doesn't necessarily lead to disease, and can actually exist in a healthy
mouth free of tooth decay. Other bacteria that were also associated
with tooth decay are now considered a normal part of a healthy oral
flora. Parents are now safe to cuddle their children again. In fact, the
more the better: Babies and children need intensive contact with the
microbia carried by others to build up their own diverse microbial
communities. The more diverse, the better. But in that case, what is
actually responsible for tooth decay?

## The Ecological Plaque Hypothesis

The model that is currently accepted is called the ecological plaque
hypothesis. This explanatory model no longer fits into a children's
book narrative but it is probably the closest to the truth. Bacteria still
play a role, but one quite different from what was previously thought.
It would appear that bacteria don't cause tooth decay simply by being
present. They only participate in the process when they are given the
opportunity to as a result of a number of factors. Rather than being
caused by individual bacteria, it is now believed that tooth decay
happens when there is an imbalance in the ecological system of the
mouth. In other words, this happens when the composition of the
bacterial community changes to our detriment or when the natural
repair systems in the mouth are overridden. This happens, for example:

1. If the pH value of the saliva and within the biofilm drops too
   low too often, or if our organism is repeatedly exposed to
   blood sugar fluctuations caused by constant sugar spikes.

2. If acid-forming bacteria are too numerous.
3. If there is too little saliva flowing into the mouth or its chemical composition is disrupted to such an extent that it can no longer balance out acid attacks and give the teeth the nutrients they need.
4. If other factors such as chronic inflammation or poor dental restorations disrupt and permanently change the microbial composition.

What we generally refer to as a hole in the tooth, dentists call a lesion. In general the same thing happens on the surface of the teeth as when we use vinegar to descale the kettle: The acid dissolves minute particles from the solid surface. Normally our saliva is able to neutralize the acid and replenish the teeth with minerals. Tooth decay does not normally progress steadily; it is a dynamic process of mineral loss and recovery. If the phases of demineralization are more frequent and longer than the replenishing phases, the lesion will expand. The essential factor that repeatedly shifts the climate in our mouths toward demineralization is our diet. Everyone knows that sugar is bad for our teeth. But we now know better than before how our teeth are affected by sugar.

## From Sweet to Sour

If we do not offer our teeth anything else, our oral bacteria behave very frugally and feed mainly on what our saliva offers them, such as glycoproteins contained in the pellicle. The bacteria metabolize them, transforming them into lactic acid, acetic acid, and propionic acid. But this is no great drama, as the buffer system in saliva can balance this type of acid quite quickly; even in an advanced biofilm, a neutral environment can prevail. As soon as fermentable carbohydrates, such as sugar, fruit, or lactose, appear, glycoproteins are quickly forgotten and certain bacteria start digging into the sugar like there's no tomorrow. The acid that they subsequently release is much more corrosive than when they only consume glycoproteins. Within three minutes of consuming the sugar, the pH in the saliva drops to a relatively low

## When Things Really Turn Sour . . .

There are certain types of tooth decay that bacteria are not at all responsible for; these arise as a direct result of acidity. This is what dentists refer to as erosion. These acids are not metabolic products of bacteria, but may arise as the result of acidic drinks, for example, such as orange juice and cola. They can also arise as the result of acid reflux or vomiting. People who suffer from acid reflux or eating disorders are therefore particularly susceptible to this type of tooth decay. A high level of acidity is very important, for splitting proteins and other tasks. But when stomach acid comes into contact with other tissues as a result of digestive problems, it can cause serious damage.

level and only returns to a normal level after twenty to thirty minutes. But bacteria don't only digest sugar; they also use its molecules to build polymers, chemicals that help them to latch onto things and entrench themselves better.

While some groups of bacteria in our mouths get some benefits from sugar that help them to survive, others cannot metabolize sugars at all, and even die when there is an excess of sugar in their environment. Others die because of the pH value. There are certain bacteria that need a neutral pH to be able to grow and are extremely sensitive to acid. Many bacteria that make up a healthy flora can only tolerate low pH levels for a short time. If the acid levels stay low for any length of time, they become inhibited or simply die. Our food can be partly responsible for this, but so can artificial built-in dental materials. In this kind of environment, the bacteria that tolerate and form acid soon outnumber the others and produce more substances that drain minerals from tooth enamel. Just like other ecosystems, our oral and intestinal flora remain healthy for as long as they are diverse. An imbalance is always a bad thing, as we see in our environment when the ecology is disrupted by environmental destruction, which makes life difficult for certain species. The same goes for our own organism.

So the film of bacteria in our mouths is not harmful per se. It only transforms into cariogenic plaque when sugar or other factors are added into the mix, because this allows the environment to remain constantly acidic. Lesions can also progress faster in the absence of the protective properties of saliva. Treatment for tooth decay is therefore no longer primarily concerned with tracking individual, presumably pathogenic microorganisms, but with correcting the chronic

## Tooth Decay Is Curable

To the naked eye tooth decay is first visible not as a dark hole but as a white spot, also known as a chalk stain. The spot appears lighter than the rest of the tooth because demineralized areas of enamel have different visual characteristics than mineralized, which means it reflects the light hitting it differently. This stage is what dentists refer to as caries incipiens and does not require intervention with a drill as was formerly thought to be the case. Tooth decay generally progresses slowly—over a period of months and years—and is reversible in this early stage. Caries incipiens can be stopped—or as dentists say, arrested—if the abnormal imbalance in the mouth can be reversed. My belief is that the tooth should first be observed and that over time, the conditions that caused the lesion should be neutralized and the phases of mineralization should be supported through the supply of the required nutrients. At this stage the tooth is still able to remineralize itself from within. Drilling early on will always destroy healthy enamel and lead to a cycle of drilling and refilling.

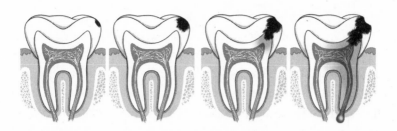

**Figure 1.3.** Tooth decay doesn't happen overnight: the various stages of tooth decay.

imbalance first and foremost, by reducing demineralizing factors and helping the remineralization process along.

We have control over many of these elements ourselves. Everything we eat either strengthens the bacteria that keep us healthy, or makes life easier for those that have a tendency to attack us. The foods we eat determine whether we support the friendly or hostile bacteria and whether we allow the peaceful varieties to spread or make way for their acid-forming counterparts. Bacteria are abundant in our mouths, which is not something we should be trying to change. We can decide for ourselves whether they harm us or not.

### Case Study: Weston Price and the Significance of Nutrition

At the turn of the twentieth century, there was a dentist I would call a legend living and working in the United States. His name was Weston Price. He was extraordinary in many ways, but if it came to picking out just one thing, it would have to be his ability to think in a broader context. Decades before science had adapted to the ecological plaque hypothesis, Price could not comprehend that individual bacteria could be responsible for the flood of patients he was receiving in his dental practice with destroyed teeth and tooth misalignments. But Price wasn't just observing a huge increase in dental disease; he was also witnessing the worsening physical condition of society in general. More and more people were becoming frail, suffering from cardiovascular disease, cancer, arthritis, or joint and back pain due to scoliosis and misalignment. Price guessed that there was a connection and subsequently devoted his life to finding out what it was. His suspicion was that the cause of the enormous increase in both dental and physical illness was to be found in our eating habits. Industrialization and technological advances had, for the first time, given people access to refined sugar, ground white flour, and artificially mass-produced products. Food was now easier to obtain and prepare, but Price guessed that people were paying the price for this new convenience. He set out to find proof that the diseases people were contracting in their mouths were primarily determined by what we eat and that the same factors not only destroy our teeth, but also have an impact on the health of our entire bodies.

In other words, Weston Price was probably the first biologically minded dental surgeon. He began to study the chemical composition of food in his laboratory and developed the theory that industrial products lacked many of the nutrients that are essential to oral and general health. And he didn't just research what was lacking in the nutrition of his own country; he also went on years' worth of expeditions to other cultures. He traveled through Africa, sailed to Australia, Peru, New Zealand, and the Polynesian islands, hiked through North America, Canada, to the North Pole, and visited farmers in the Swiss mountains. When he selected his destinations, a couple of criteria were particularly important to him: First, he wanted to find populations that were as isolated and primordial as possible. Second, he wanted to document changes as a result of contact with the rest of civilization.

Wherever Price went, he made the same observation: Wherever people were eating the same way their ancestors did and had hardly any contact with modern nutritional practices, their teeth were not only healthy, but also straight. Their jaws provided enough space for all their teeth; they had broad nostrils and breathed through their noses. Their physiques were generally strong. He didn't find people who performed meticulous oral hygiene or regularly used dental floss. On the contrary: Apart from a few sticks used to clean their teeth, most of the people he met didn't have any specific dental hygiene regimes. The teeth of most of the people he encountered were almost completely covered in starchy foods, and they made no special effort to clean them. Despite all this, they did not have any signs of tooth decay; in fact they seemed to be immune to it.

What they lacked in oral hygiene, they made up for elsewhere: Primordial diets were generally natural, were untreated, and, according to Price's analysis, contained many more fat-soluble vitamins and had a higher calcium content, as well as many other important minerals. The industrial revolution had shifted the balance in the oral microbia. Today it is believed that the diversity in our mouths has decreased dramatically in comparison with those who lived as hunter-gatherers. At the same time, today's diets deprive human beings of the important nutrients they need to fight tooth decay from within. We have become accustomed to seeing teeth as lifeless objects. But they have a lively, dynamic core that nourishes and maintains them. The pulp, the innermost core of the tooth, is permanently flooded and rinsed with liquid from the body. If our body chemistry is out of balance as a result of nutrition, our teeth will always suffer. Constant blood sugar spikes damage the tooth not only from the outside, but from the inside, too. This is because high blood sugar levels choke the supply of oxygen and nutrients and weaken the natural supply and defense mechanisms of the teeth and gums. A very similar process takes place when our bodies are deficient in certain nutrients. The pulp can sometimes literally wither away as a result. Scientists have found that a vitamin $D_3$ deficiency can have a drastic effect on the pulp that can be seen on an X-ray: The pulp appears much narrower and less swollen.[14]

Dentin and enamel largely consist of the minerals calcium and phosphorus. These can only be stored in the organism with the help of vitamin D in the teeth and bones. An optimal supply hardens the teeth and promotes the formation of new dentin. The more nutrients the pulp is able to supply, the more nourishment the tooth receives and the stronger its immune system. So our teeth are very much alive, and they need a well-balanced intake of minerals, vitamins, and proteins to stay strong and healthy.

Although it is very clear that diet has a huge impact on dental health and the health of the organism in general, too little attention is paid to the topic of medicine, and dental medicine too often remains the focus. Other than halfhearted warnings not to snack too much, there are no other real guidelines. The industrial influence on the

## Cavities Have Competition . . .

While tooth decay is now on the decline, particularly in children, another tooth disease is becoming more common. Its rather complicated name is molar incisor hypomineralization, or MIH for short. They are sometimes simply referred to as chalk teeth—a name that unfortunately describes the substance of the affected teeth quite well. The first signs of MIH are often cream-colored or brown spots on the humps of the molars (back teeth) or incisors (front teeth). Teeth become painful and sensitive to the touch, and no wonder: The patches are a sign that the structure of the normally rock-hard enamel is significantly destroyed. The affected teeth can become so soft that they feel like chalk and sometimes simply crumble under strain. MIH affects up to 10 percent of children in Germany. Although that is a significant number, researchers and clinicians still don't know enough about the causes of the disease or how to treat it correctly.

MIH remains an enigma for experts. Nevertheless, the name gives us an idea of the nature of the beast: a

production of our food is now much greater than when Weston Price began seeking the cause of the illnesses he was observing.

Nutrition is a central component in my concept of dentistry. I'm convinced that medicine should always guide people toward healthy eating habits. (See "The Healing Power of Nutrition" on page 126.)

## Iatrogenic Factors: When Dentists Are Responsible for Dental Problems

The relationship between dentist and patient seems to be clearly regulated: The patient does something wrong, like getting tooth hypomineralization, or shortage of nutrients. Several factors have been proposed as potential causes: MIH is associated with celiac disease (gluten intolerance), a disease that prevents the body from absorbing enough nutrients as a result of a permanently irritated intestinal lining. Other suspects include foods that cause inflammations in the gastrointestinal tract and destroy the intestinal mucosa, causing issues with nutrient uptake. These include lectins and agglutinins from wheat or other cereals. Other studies indicate that the plasticizer bisphenol A may play a role. In experiments on rats, the rodents developed porous teeth when fed with the substance.

Other potential culprits include antibiotic treatments in early childhood, the influence of environmental toxins such as dioxin, and infectious diseases contracted by the mother during pregnancy. My recommendation for those affected is to start by checking levels of vitamin $D_3$, which helps deliver calcium to teeth and bones along with its key co-factors, magnesium and vitamin $K_2$.

decay or some other dental problem, and the dentist repairs the damage. What we rarely realize is that sometimes, the dentist is the one who causes the problem. In medicine we sometimes hear iatrogenic factors being mentioned in hushed voices. Yet these factors are not all that uncommon. Unfortunately, conventional dentistry not only solves problems, it sometimes also causes them. The wrong diet does have a significant influence on changes in the microflora in the mouth, and therefore on any initial damage that occurs. But many dental interventions can further aggravate the problem. This is not necessarily because the dentist has worked badly; it's just that any dental work carried out changes the conditions in the mouth completely. This should be kept in mind, especially in the cases of the following common treatments.

### Mind the Gap: Why Fillings Are Not Always Useful

If a tooth has a cavity, a dentist will remove the affected tooth substance and fill the hole. Of course, they will take care that the material adheres well to the tooth and that the hole is properly sealed. Many fillings, however, eventually begin to show what are known as marginal gaps, which are gaps around the edges of fillings that are sometimes microscopically small. The gaps alone are not enough to provide hideouts for bacteria to escape oral hygiene and multiply zealously. Rather, the composition of the bacterial ratio changes, which can provide favorable conditions for the next cavity or the progression of chronic gingivitis. Drilling teeth too early on can also damage enamel. This is why it's always better to wait in the case of initial tooth decay and concentrate on changing the conditions triggering the problem. The vicious cycle caused by fillings starts with the first filling. The different factors to take into account with regard to different materials are described in detail in chapter 2; see "Teeth and Toxicology" on page 67.

Often fillings are overused in treating tooth decay; dentists have simply become too generous with them. If the filling material reaches below the gum line, pathogenic anaerobes can spread, which are microorganisms that can live in an oxygen-free environment and change the entire climate within the mouth. This also happens if a dentist does not pay enough attention to a tiny area in the mouth when fitting a crown: the biological width.

### Biological Width: A Matter of Millimeters

Even today, many crowns contain a certain proportion of metal, especially in the hidden posterior region of the mouth, and are slipped on top of teeth that are discolored or have been treated at the root. The crown may look nice, but it can quickly develop an unsightly black edge. Of course, every dentist wants the work to look good afterward, so they try to push the crown edge as far as possible under the gum line. But in the case of root canal treatment

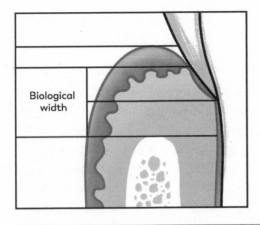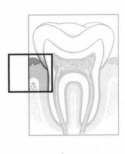

Figure 1.4. Biological width: The longevity of crowns and implants is determined in this tiny area.

in particular, this is nothing but a dangerous masquerade; it is no longer performed in biological dentistry. If the edge of the crown is set too deep, it often causes damage to a very sensitive area known as the biological width.

Biological width plays a decisive role in determining whether a crown or implant will last. This is because injuries in the mouth mean the gums are exposed to constant, localized irritation. The tissue can become inflamed; bone loss is accelerated and eventually leads to tooth loss or implants. Luckily, many dentists (especially those specializing in aesthetic surgery) already work with ceramic restorations, which are the same color as teeth and therefore do not have to be hidden under the gums. Furthermore, significantly less plaque accumulates on full ceramic restorations and ceramic implants.

### The Key Role of Filling Materials

Even fillings that are supposed to repair the tooth can cause problems, sometimes simply because they produce a surface that is rougher than a natural tooth. Often they also contain substances that permanently disturb the oral flora. For example, metals—mercury in particular— are antibacterial. Sometimes this fact is sold as an advantage. But the bactericidal action of the metal does not distinguish between

## A Tiny Mistake with Big Consequences

Our mouths are the key to the structure of the rest of our bodies. Whether or not our skeleton and its supporting muscles are symmetrical and straight depends on the condition of our mouths. The positioning of our eyes and teeth are directly related. The eyes of every mammal are reflexively focused on the horizon (the tonic labyrinthine reflex), and even the smallest changes to the position of the teeth can lead to an imbalance in the structure. Often a change in the range of micrometers is enough to trigger the body to try to compensate for the change using regulating mechanisms in the muscle and ligament structure and by shifting connective tissue interfaces in the skull area. This usually manifests itself as tension in the deep neck muscles, but it can also have an effect on the shoulder and pelvic area over time. In the long term this can lead to misalignments and bad posture. Anyone looking for the cause of these symptoms should start by checking the functionality of the mouth. Sometimes a filling that's too high or crowns that are not properly ground are enough to trigger these issues. What's more, chronic stressors in the mouth and throat area can often lead to tension in the upper cervical spine, as problems stemming from the mouth spread directly to this area via the nervous system. Almost all patients who come to me suffer from neck tension. In 80 percent of cases, the cause can be found in their mouths.

beneficial and harmful microorganisms. Built-in metals can permanently damage the oral flora.

A normal, diverse variety of bacterial flora is good for us. But when it changes, it becomes dangerous. If pathogenic bacteria take over,

## Fillings:
## Sometimes They're Just Not All There

Giving a tooth a filling or crown is no guarantee that tooth decay will not return in the future. It is precisely these "repaired" areas that are at risk of further lesions. When tooth decay appears on the edge of a filling or crown, this is known as secondary tooth decay. Secondary tooth decay is most commonly caused by fissures between the tooth and filling or crowns that are not completely sealed.

they not only wreak havoc in our mouths but also try to cross an important boundary.

## Gingiva: A Sensitive Issue

Between the teeth and gums lies a thin border that marks an important barrier in our bodies: the border between interior and exterior. As soon as a bite of food disappears from our mouths, most people assume it is simply "inside" us. Strictly speaking, however, this is not the case. Our entire mouth is covered in what is known as the squamous epithelium, which is the anatomical term for outer skin. Foreign substances and microorganisms cannot get inside us without crossing this barrier. The border between the tooth and gums—also known as the gingiva—is the part of the body where this can happen more easily than anywhere else, as this area forms a sort of ditch or recess.

Bacteria are in their element in this kind of environment.

The body makes sure that they don't get very far, however, because the gums usually cling very strongly to the teeth. The gums can also be imagined as a very tight cuff that is stretched around our teeth. This not only fixes our teeth very firmly in the root bed, but also protects the delicate boundary between the inside of our bodies and

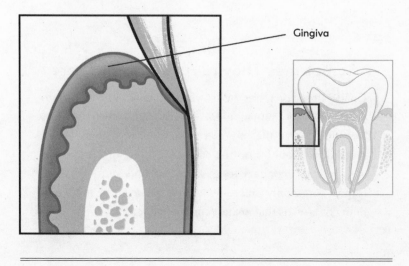

Gingiva

**Figure 1.5.** Healthy gums form a solid unit with the tooth.

our environment. Nevertheless, some microorganisms still manage to slip through due to micro-injuries that occur when chewing or brushing teeth. If the oral flora is in balance and we are otherwise healthy, this isn't usually a problem. But serious issues can arise if the composition of the microorganisms is imbalanced and our immune systems are no longer able to defend this sensitive border.

When bacteria gain the upper hand in our mouths and trigger inflammatory processes, the border becomes weaker. Inflammation causes swelling, which in turn loosens the tissue and makes it easier for microorganisms to occupy the area. At this point even doctors resort to military language and call this phenomenon a bacterial invasion.

We often don't realize that a war is raging in our gums. Unfortunately we can barely notice anything in our bathroom mirrors or when we flash a smile at someone. At most the gums might be slightly red and swollen, which most people don't notice. These signs would not escape the rigorous, knowledgeable gaze of a dental expert, however, who would label these symptoms "gingivitis" once a certain level of inflammation is reached. If the patient deals with the cause (such as a bad filling or tartar), pays attention to their diet, and cleans their teeth well, the problem can usually be fixed within in a short space of time.

## Receding Gums

Sometimes people find that their gums begin to recede at the root of the tooth. It looks like the tooth has become slightly longer because more of it is visible. The main reason for this is usually incorrect, aggressive oral hygiene. In other words: rough, horizontal brushing. A change in brushing technique and being gentler with the gums is usually enough to get this under control. Making more circular motions with a toothbrush is often enough for the gums to recover. Other factors that can cause gum damage are problems such as grinding and clenching. Both of these can result from a misalignment in the jaw, but also from chronic irritation of the autonomic nervous system from metals, inflammation, or other root canal treatments in the mouth.

If the problem is not dealt with, the inflammation progresses to the next level: periodontitis.

## Periodontitis: A Threat to the Whole Body

When microorganisms overstep a critical limit, the consequences are disastrous on many levels. The first consequences are at the local level, given that inflammation now has access to a very valuable part of our periodontal apparatus known as Sharpey's fibers, and begins to destroy it. These are very special, strong fibers that are only found in this specific part of the body. They are very important when it comes to ensuring that our teeth are firmly anchored in the jaw. Most people imagine that teeth are fused with the jawbone, but this would restrict the flexibility of our teeth. Teeth are not as fixed as we may think. Each is essentially loosely suspended in the periodontium, and for good reason: This way, teeth spring and slide slightly when we chew.

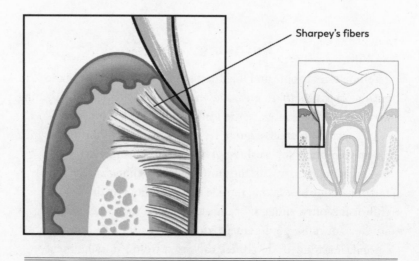

**Figure 1.6.** Sharpey's fibers provide grip and flexibility for our teeth.

If you clench your teeth together tightly and wiggle them back and forth a little, you can feel this flexibility quite well. This is not a sign that your teeth are too loose; in fact, they need this flexibility so that they can give way if we unexpectedly bite into something hard. Without a certain level of flexibility, our teeth would become damaged much more often.

Periodontitis makes short work of destroying this tissue irreversibly. Once Sharpey's fibers are destroyed by inflammation, the tooth soon loses its grip. It first becomes loose, then falls out completely. Sadly this isn't just a horror story; in fact it happens quite frequently. Tooth decay has clearly been on the decline in recent years, but around 70 percent of adults in Germany between the ages of thirty-five and fifty and over 80 percent of senior citizens suffer from periodontal disease. From the age of thirty-five, more teeth are lost as a result of inflammation than tooth decay. From a certain age onward, tooth loss can therefore mainly be attributed to periodontitis.

Although periodontitis has become frighteningly widespread, many people still know too little about it and, more important, about its disastrous consequences. Presumably this is due to the fact that periodontitis is just as difficult to spot as gingivitis under certain circumstances.

In both cases the red tissue surrounding the tooth doesn't always look like a cause for concern. But if we were to look deeper into our anatomy, we would think differently, because periodontitis hides in the depths of the tooth that are invisible to the naked eye. If you were to put the average surface area of affected tissue together, the resulting wound would be the size of the palm of a human hand.

No one would simply carry on with their lives as normal if they had a wound this size, nor try to downplay or ignore its severity. We would probably want to make sure that the wound is properly treated and able to heal. And yet in the case of periodontitis, the problem is sadly often left for years. Even if we ignore it, our immune system will not. Periodontitis is a huge burden on our immune system because it constantly has to deal with the dangerous inflammatory substances it produces and the stress this puts the nervous system under. It is one of the long-term, chronic inflammatory issues that we now know can directly or indirectly trigger many other diseases. Furthermore, like any other inflammation, periodontitis tends to progress—and not just within the mouth. When the border between the inside and outside world is crossed, a whole new world awaits microorganisms: the body.

From here, they can take over our cardiovascular system or create the right conditions for Alzheimer's or diabetes.

Periodontitis is a disease of the mouth, and as such is primarily treated there. But I see it as a systemic disease and also treat it as

## Why Did Sailors' Teeth Fall Out?

Years ago, sailors would spend months on the ocean with no access to fresh food. A lack of vitamin C in particular soon manifested itself in dental problems: Gums would begin to bleed, and teeth would loosen until, finally, they fell out completely. The reason for this is that the body needs vitamin C to make and store collagen, which makes up the fibers that anchor our teeth firmly in the periodontium.

## Two Names, One Disease

Periodontitis continues to be referred to by its former name, parodontosis. However, only the term with the suffix *-itis*, usually used for inflammatory diseases, is correct. This name change alone demonstrates how much our knowledge of gum disease has changed. It used to be understood as a common disease of the periodontium, but we now know that it's the result of chronic inflammation.

such. This is because, generally speaking, the problem cannot be solved in the mouth or with better toothbrushing techniques alone. Anyone who has been suffering from periodontitis will confirm this. Any treatment should involve allowing the body to defend itself. It is therefore not enough to treat periodontitis in the mouth only, but also via one of the supersystems in our bodies: the immune system.

# Teeth and the Immune System

If we were able to see our immune system, even a short trip to the supermarket would seem as complex as a visit from the head of state. There's an escort to protect us from our surroundings; snipers are positioned on surrounding rooftops; bodyguards, SWAT teams, and other special forces are lined up in all directions muttering instructions to one another by radio, ready to intervene promptly should a suspicious object get too close. In the eyes of the immune system, such trivial matters as breathing, drinking a cappuccino, or lying under a tree in the grass are enough to trigger a red alert in our bodies. Because every particle we come into contact with—whether it touches our skin, penetrates our lungs, or is swallowed—is regarded by our immune system as foreign or hostile. The immune system touches and examines everything suspiciously before either waving it through, or standing to attention then intervening should the intruder not be welcome after all. Our immune system isn't only required when we're ill; it's constantly in use. It has an army of around ten billion immune cells and hundreds of millions more antibodies at its disposal. Each of these special cells is invisible to the naked eye, but if you were to stack them all in one pile, they would produce a mass weighing over four pounds. They are not usually found together, however, as our immune cells are distributed throughout the whole body. There are main centers in the intestine, spleen, and bone marrow, as well as external centers in the lymph nodes.

The immune system is one of the most complex systems in the body, but many of its basic functions are easy to understand if we compare them to Pac-Man. That's right, Pac-Man, the legendary computer game from the 1980s, invented at a time when graphics and manufacturers' imaginations yielded little more than a tiny half circle wandering through a maze, opening and closing its mouth to eat points. Our immune system has certain participants that essentially work in the same way as Pac-Man. They're called macrophages and they protect us by rendering harmless anything they deem as foreign, poisonous, or inflammatory, simply by eating it up. Biology is sometimes terribly complicated, but sometimes it can be gloriously simple.

Unlike Pac-Man, however, macrophages have an additional special function: They release what are known as immunocytokines—messenger substances that stimulate other parts of the immune system into action, when reinforcements are needed. Many of these messenger substances have long, obscure names such as TNF alpha, interleukin 1 beta, or NF kappa B. Despite their complicated names, they tackle things that we are all familiar with: the pus-filled blister that begins to form on the finger when we get a splinter, or the fever we experience when we get a virus. In other words: Immunocytokines trigger inflammation. We can be sure they are at work from the moment we say to ourselves: *I'm not feeling well, I think I'll go and have a lie down.*

So while we're lying in bed feeling sick, our organism is dancing to the beat of the immunocytokines and following their orders. A sick animal doesn't go to hunt, and neither does our organism, because suddenly the immune system needs all its available energy. This is why the messenger substances in the immune system also flick the switch to "catabolic" when we are not well. Catabolic is the opposite of anabolic, which is the condition that bodybuilders strive for because it allows their muscles to grow. In a catabolic condition, on the other hand, the body begins to break down. This is not a time for the body to store nutrients, amino acids, and minerals; they need to be available for the immune system to use. This is why we often feel a little groggy once we get over an infection. Our immune system has allocated itself a substantial proportion of the energy, nutrients, and other substances it needs to put in the extra work required for fighting the infection and getting us back on our feet again.

## Superfoods for Super Health

When we start to get ill, nutrition is crucial, and it's important not to be tempted to eat rubbish just because we're not feeling well. The organism is running at full speed and doesn't need to waste any extra energy trying to compensate for the wrong foods. On the contrary, this is precisely the right time to be giving our bodies the kind of foods that act as medicine: superfoods.

# Silent and Deadly: Chronic Inflammation

Acute inflammation is therefore quite useful and can help us. It becomes problematic, however, if it isn't able to do its job quickly enough. Immunocytokines help us out a lot in the short term, but they start to do more harm than good if they are constantly activated. The processes that take place when we have chronic inflammation and acute inflammation are essentially the same, only they occur at a constant, low level in the case of chronic. We might feel ill, but only a little. We might feel like we're getting a fever, but it never really breaks out. Our metabolism is running constantly on low, while our insulin and fat metabolisms begin to change. The muscle and bone tissues begin to break down and store fatty tissues. All of these processes happen at what is known as the subclinical level, which means we don't realize they are happening. This is also known as silent inflammation. It might not cause any pain or knock us off our feet, but this is precisely what makes it so dangerous: It has a long-term unseen influence on our organism and sends it the wrong signals. If you wanted to knock out a boxer in the ring, you could either do it by punching them really hard once, or by delivering a series of small blows to their knee.

The way we currently live our lives, our immune systems have become like this boxer in the ring, being attacked from all sides. Many aspects of our daily lives put our bodies at risk of inflammation: foods

## Dead Teeth Don't Scream

Whenever we buy a new perfume, the fragrance seems very strong at first. A few days later, it's not as strong, until at some point we feel like we have to keep spraying more and more perfume to be able to smell it at all. This is because the body down-regulates the smell receptors that perceive fragrances when they are too strong for it. A similar thing happens with our pain receptors. In a way, chronic disease is just our bodies getting lazy or becoming accustomed to certain conditions. Unfortunately, this sometimes results in cysts the size of peas forming at the root of a dead tooth. If the patient does not feel any pain, a dentist might suggest leaving the tooth, despite the presence of a chronic lesion.

full of white flour and sugar, pesticides, and environmental toxins. But stress can also keep our immune systems constantly activated. In the Western world chronic diseases such as cardiovascular disease, diabetes, allergies, autoimmune diseases, and inflammatory bowel diseases have been on the increase for years. All of these diseases are caused by chronic, subclinical activation of the immune system, often in the form of chronic inflammation or stress. The bottom line is that for many people, the cause of chronic inflammation can be found directly in the mouth, where it activates the immune and nervous systems twenty-four hours a day.

Unfortunately, these kinds of issues are so often overlooked because dentists are trained to respond to one symptom: acute pain. Chronic inflammations and diseases do not come with any pain symptoms, because the body has long become accustomed to its condition and down-regulated the corresponding receptors.

But which chronic diseases do come with pain symptoms? Does diabetes hurt? High blood pressure? Do those with an underactive thyroid or depression feel pain? Taking into account health as a whole, it is irresponsible to tolerate any kind of chronic inflammation—and consequently, chronic stress for the body—regardless of where it's located. If the aim is to be as healthy as possible, these factors have to be taken into account.

## Root Canals: The Root of All Evil

Sometimes, all it takes is an unfortunate fall or a sports accident for a tooth to be shaken or shifted in such a way that the blood vessels that connect the tooth's interior with the rest of the organism are simply torn away. Soon the tooth meets the same fate as any other tissue that is cut off from the blood supply: It dies. In a tooth this primarily affects the pulp—the vital internal core. The effect of this pulp loss on the other layers of the tooth quickly becomes apparent: The tooth becomes brittle and begins to discolor. It stands out between other, healthy teeth because it turns either yellow or gray. This is the first sign for some people that the tooth is dead. Others realize when the dentist performs a vitality test. If the tooth no longer reacts to a cold stimulus, the pulp is very likely to be dead. A tooth that has died as the result of an accident often does so without making itself known.

Teeth more commonly die because bacteria have made their way to the inside of the tooth as a result of tooth decay—and this is anything but painless. When this happens, the pulp becomes inflamed, which causes both hellish pain and often, the characteristic swollen cheek. Anyone who has been putting off a trip to the dentist will suddenly be champing at the bit to finally see someone. Radiating pain is a typical symptom at this stage, as is biting pain—and indeed the feeling of having been hit in the mouth with a jackhammer.

The standard treatment for a tooth with a dead or inflamed pulp is known as root canal treatment. Root canals are a wonderful thing in theory, but in practice they can be a disaster for the patient's health. Ever since dentists began performing them, all sorts of problems have started to arise. This is not due to a lack of ability on the part of dentists, but to the undeniable fact that the roots of teeth are unpredictable. The root canals of teeth are never the same. From the outside,

## Odontoblasts: Paramedics for the Teeth

Our teeth aren't only connected to the body as a whole; they also have their own immune systems. When bacteria get dangerously close to the inside of the tooth, certain cells known as odontoblasts register the invasion early on and come in like specially trained paramedics. First of all, before initiating any rescue measures, they raise the alarm with the immune system by setting in motion inflammatory processes. If tooth decay progresses quickly, they respond with what is known as tubular sclerosis. In nonmedical terms: They petrify. This petrification process is not just a resigned stiffening. It is an attempt to quickly close the tiny entrances that lead to the sensitive pulp and stop bacteria from advancing. At the same time, the odontoblasts produce irritation dentin, which is released to bother the bacteria. Once we know a bit more about the heroic battles odontoblasts are constantly fighting to protect our teeth, it is very difficult to continue viewing teeth as inanimate chewing tools.

it's almost impossible to determine which direction they grow in and how they branch out, or how many roots a tooth even has. The hidden part of the tooth is always a surprise for dentists.

Front teeth, which usually only have one canal, are fairly easy to size up. Molars, on the other hand, have three or four roots. They sometimes look like the root system of a young plant that has been pulled from the ground what with all their branches and numerous accessory canals.

At the beginning of the twentieth century, we hardly knew anything at all about the versatility of tooth roots. Dentist Walter Hess had the idea of cataloging them so that dentists would know in the future the number of roots each type of tooth has. In an extremely

## Eye for an Eye, Tooth for a Tooth

Our canine teeth have particularly long roots—in fact, these roots reach all the way up to the eye socket, so it's no wonder canines are sometimes referred to as the eyetooth. Inflammation in this area is sometimes discovered when a patient experiences intense pressure pain underneath the eye. Usually, these are the last teeth we lose because their roots are so strong. They are located in the same place as the fangs of a predatory animal. Animals die if they lose these teeth because they are no longer able to hunt their prey.

## Everything Must Go

One hundred years ago a standard was established for root canal treatment: "What you get out of the tooth is more important than what you put in." This is because any dead pulp tissue left behind is perfect fodder for bacteria, and also because the body will try to break it down itself, which leads to the production of toxic degradation products. In every other field of medicine, the removal of dead tissue is always a priority.

comprehensive examination and dissection of twenty-eight hundred teeth, he did not find the commonality he was looking for, but instead a vast range of different tooth roots.

Practically every tooth has a completely individual root system. Some come in strange shapes, some have numerous protrusions; some are curved in a C-shape and others elliptic. Even the front

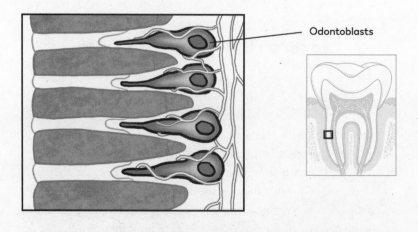

**Figure 2.1.** Odontoblasts protect our teeth from the inside.

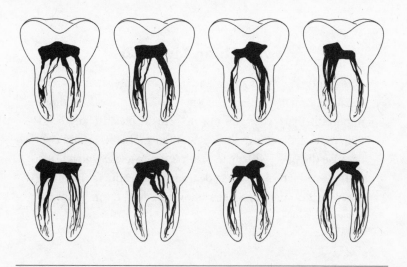

**Figure 2.2.** The root canals of molars come in a huge variety.

teeth, which were previously thought to have only a single root, sometimes revealed a full fringe of roots beneath their tips. Walter Hess's catalog demonstrated what an incredible variety of tooth roots there is in existence. To this day his work is considered ground-breaking and has even stood the test of modern methods such as

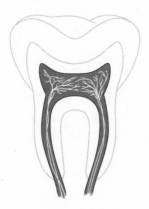

**Figure 2.3.** The pulp, also known as the tooth nerve, fills up the inside of our teeth.

high-resolution microcomputer tomographies, which all confirm what he documented in 1917: Tooth roots are just as individual and versatile as people.

Every dentist knows that a complete removal of the pulp and cleaning and filling of a root canal is nigh on impossible due to this complicated anatomy. This can be described as a mechanical limitation. That said, dentists now have new ways of mapping out the canals and their branches as accurately as possible. Some dentists work with a surgical microscope that magnifies up to 30x and provides highly effective illumination of the area in question. Of course, it's also important to take an X-ray to get an idea of where everything is. But some root canals are not visible at all. What's more, the older a patient gets, the more difficult it becomes to locate everything, because root canals grow increasingly narrow with age. Even if every single branch is located, there still remains a part of the tooth root that is inaccessible despite any sophisticated technology we may use: the dentinal tubules.

Technically the pulp is considered to be a separate entity from the two other types of tooth tissue, but in reality it is tightly interwoven with them. The pulp and dentin form a biological functional unit, which is aptly named the pulp-dentin complex. The two tissues

## The Problem with Time Pressure

The low success rate of many root canal treatments undoubtedly has a lot to do with health insurance policies. These policies deem a root filling sufficient if it reaches the apical third of the root canal. This means the root is not completely filled and it's deemed acceptable for dead tissue to remain in the tooth. What's more, a thorough root canal treatment is a very time-intensive procedure. It takes at least three to four hours to properly treat a molar with four roots. This is simply not covered by statutory health insurance.

are connected via countless delicate little channels. These channels provide the dentin with nourishment, and connect the exterior roots with the interior nerves, which determine whether the tooth's own immune system has to resort to defense measures. These tubules are incredibly delicate but also incredibly numerous—there are between thirty thousand and seventy-five thousand per square millimeter. If they were all laid out in a row, they would be more than half a mile in length, per root. This part of a tooth can't be removed, cleaned, or filled. A root canal treatment is therefore a bit like trying to clean the canal system of Venice by only treating the water of the Grand Canal.

## The Consequences of Root Canal Treatments

Around eight million root canal treatments are carried out every year in Germany alone. A root canal is a very effective treatment method for acute pain. As soon as a dentist has removed the living interior part of the tooth, the agonizing pain is relieved. In the long term, however, root canal treatments always lead to complications. Sixty percent of follow-up root canal treatments are carried out due to roots that have not been completely filled in. It's sometimes possible for

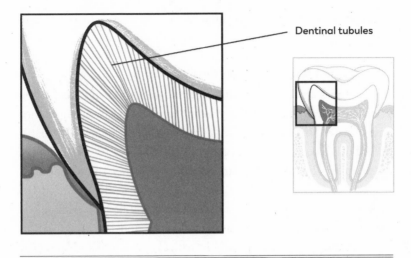

Figure 2.4. Even if the pulp could be completely removed during a root canal treatment, no dental tools would be able to reach the extremely delicate dentinal tubules.

a dentist to miss part of the root canal because it's not visible, and sometimes the root canal is not filled to the end because there is a bend or kink in it. In any case, there is no way of accessing accessory canals and dentinal tubules. Every tooth that has undergone a root canal treatment is colonized by bacteria over time. Sometimes this happens quickly, sometimes over a longer period of time.

The risks and consequences of a root canal treatment are not addressed in dentistry studies. But like any other dentist at the beginning of their career, I always felt very uncomfortable carrying out root canal treatments: Some teeth are so badly inflamed, porous, or mushy, and smell so bad, that intuition alone can tell you the treatment will not suffice on a long-term basis. I only became aware later on through my own research on the subject that there is a long history of controversy in dentistry when it comes to root canal treatments.

Tooth roots/canals are the perfect cavity for microorganisms to hide in. Because of their extremely remote location, they host many anaerobes—bacteria that cope very well in environments low in oxygen. If a dead tooth is colonized with bacteria, this becomes a problem for all of the areas around this tooth because these bacteria love to spread. But first they have to get past the immune system.

## Case Study: Under Fire from the Outset

For centuries there was only one option for dead or inflamed teeth: They fell victim to pliers. This meant the problem disappeared, but unfortunately, the tooth did, too. Finally, when the focus of dentistry shifted to preservation—the conservation and reparation of teeth—people were able to keep their teeth, but suddenly clinical pictures started to pile up that made dentists skeptical. At the beginning of the twentieth century, many physicians already had connections to the work of their colleagues in dentistry. Around 1911 Englishman William Hunter expressed a highly critical opinion of and launched a virulent attack on septic dentistry. Increasing numbers of dentists began to believe that new dental treatments literally cemented bacteria and toxins in the body. Another doctor dubbed teeth that had undergone root canal treatments "a sea of sepsis under a mausoleum of gold."[1] Heart disease, arthritis, and new forms of rheumatoid arthritis, kidney inflammation, and subfebrile medical conditions were observed in patients suffering from inflamed tooth roots or jawbones. But how could a tooth be responsible for sickness in the distant heart, or swelling in the joints? Many doctors at the time devoted themselves to the study of "focal infection theory." They assumed that bacteria could gradually occupy the tissue surrounding an inflamed tooth and eventually reach the bloodstream via any other organ in the body. One dentist who was particularly devoted to researching this phenomenon was Weston Price, whom we have already encountered in this book. He carried out numerous experiments on rabbits, implanting infected teeth that had received root canal treatments under their skin. A large number of animals soon developed the same symptoms as the respective patients Price had removed the teeth from. Price repeated the experiments many times and got the same results over and over again.[2] If the human had an infected kidney, for example, the rabbit also suffered from kidney problems. If the patient had a problem with their heart, the rabbit would soon start to get symptoms in its own heart. Price was convinced that certain bacteria have an affinity for certain tissues and a tendency to emigrate to these tissues. Other physicians tried to explain their theories via diagnosis *ex juvantibus*, which is a Latin expression meaning "confirmation of diagnosis based on success of healing." Many doctors had observed that their patients' symptoms soon improved when the diseased teeth were removed. At the time, this was not sufficient proof for the scientific community. Today it is widely considered that bacteria from the mouth are flushed into the rest of the body and then become lodged elsewhere. Price was in fact right with his assumption at the time: In teeth that had undergone root canals for inflammation at the tip, seventy-five different strains of bacteria were found, of which certain strains have an affinity for certain tissues. Four of these species preferentially infect the heart, three the nervous system, two the kidneys and brain, and one the maxillary sinus. Each of these locations can become the next center of a new infection in the body and keep the immune system activated on a constant basis.[3]

## Cysts, Fistulas, and Inflammation of the Tooth Root

The immune system has a few tricks up its sleeve for preventing microorganisms from spreading elsewhere. Its first trick, which is most commonly seen on a tooth that has been colonized by bacteria, is a cyst. A cyst is a sac of tissue that builds up around the infection to keep it separate from the rest of the body. The sac can be filled with pus (also called leukocytes, or white blood cells)—in other words, the immune system's bacteria-fighting cells. Our body wants to get rid of pus, but with a tooth cyst that's deeply embedded in the tissue, this isn't such an easy task. That said, our bodies are clever things, so they simply build a pathway for transporting the pus out. Doctors call these pathways fistulas. They can be felt on the gum near the infected tooth as a painful bump, which soon develops a yellow cap, before finally bursting open and emptying itself. But this does not solve the problem. The body has rid itself of the thing that was bothering it, so it experiences a certain relief. But for as long as the cause of the

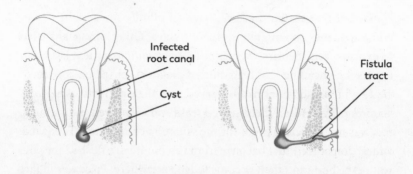

**Figure 2.5.** Inflammation of the tooth root can manifest in different ways.

problem remains present, either the capsule will fill up again or the cystic granulation tissue (taut connective tissue) will remain in the jaw as part of the chronic inflammation process and spread farther—usually destroying the surrounding bone tissue with it.

Even if a cyst with a fistula is not something we really want to have, it still gives us some reason to be happy: It's a clear indication that something is wrong, and hopefully will be enough to convince the person in question to turn to their doctor. But there are also cases in which it is not anatomically possible for a pathway to be built for transporting the pus away. In these cases a cyst at the root of the tooth can go unnoticed for a long time, grow inward, and cause a whole host of problems. Cysts that go unnoticed can become huge and grow into the jawbone, eventually destroying it. Sometimes these radicular cysts also grow in the sensitive maxillary sinus.

Another way in which the immune system responds to inflammation around teeth after root canal treatment is through ankylosis. We can think of ankylosis as a kind of prison wall. The body simply stops the metabolism process in the affected area, which causes the tissue in and around the tooth to grow very tightly, as though petrified. This creates a kind of protective wall. Ankylosis is a tough problem to treat and can sometimes take hours to deal with. It often occurs in teeth that have become particularly toxic due to metals and inflammation. But even ankylosis can go undetected for a long time, because there aren't usually any symptoms.

### Apicoectomy

When dentists discover inflammation around the root of a tooth, the common procedure is for them to carry out a rescue attempt: an apicoectomy. They might perform the procedure themselves or refer the patient to a surgeon. This is because an apicoectomy is an invasive surgical procedure. First of all, the gum is opened, then the jawbone is exposed enough so that the dentist or surgeon can access the diseased root tip, separating it from the tooth and removing it. The rest of the tooth can then stay in the jaw. An apicoectomy is a hellish operation and usually only provides temporary relief because the cause of the inflammation still remains in the body. It's a bit like responding to engine failure in a car by unscrewing the indicator light. What's more, the patient has to go through an operation that ruins the jawbone and leaves a permanent scar in the gum. In some cases, the tip of the tooth root is also sealed off with what is known as a retrograde filling or seal. This leads to allergenic or even toxic material entering the jawbone directly, without first being regulated and detoxified by the protective mechanisms in the liver. In the past amalgam was used for this procedure, which then spread throughout the jawbone and gums. It's almost impossible to remove these residues.

## NICOs: Wisdom Tooth Extraction and Its Consequences

Not everyone requires root canal treatment, of course, and it would be nice if those who don't could relax, safe in the knowledge that they are spared the huge burden of this chronic source of inflammation. Unfortunately this isn't the case. In addition to infections caused by root canal treatment, there is something else in the mouth that can cause major immunological problems. Something that often doesn't cause any localized symptoms and therefore frequently goes unrecognized. I overlooked it myself for a very long time.

So far, I have never suffered from a single cavity in my teeth; they have never needed any repair work whatsoever, so I would never have suspected that my teeth were to blame when, a few years ago, my skin broke out terribly and I suffered from a number of other symptoms, including an itchy, red rash on my forehead and cheeks. At night I was grinding my teeth like mad, my neck was always tight, my back hurt, my fingers were always falling asleep, and I frequently woke up with numb hands. I had terrible tension across my shoulders and my posture was no longer at its best, which I put down to having to sit in the dentist chair on a daily basis and tried to cure with a variety of neck pillows for sleeping at night. Having skin problems can be awful. People always bring it up. I had already learned a great deal about healthy nutrition and paid a lot of attention to what I ate. But suddenly everyone started saying: "You look rough . . . you should watch what you're eating." It was frustrating. At the time I had been working with my friend and former mentor Dr. Ulrich Volz in his clinic. One day I felt so miserable I could barely concentrate. One of our visiting colleagues insisted on carrying out kinesiologic tests on me. This involves checking the autonomic nervous system for its ability to regulate by means of what is known as a muscle test. A trained therapist is able to determine in just a few steps what the cause behind the symptom is. Since I myself am trained in ART (autonomic response testing), I had no doubts about taking this type of test.

In the end, my colleague told me that the field of disturbance was in my mouth. I could hardly believe it, and thought that if anything, the nighttime grinding would be the culprit. When we localized the disturbance field in the wisdom tooth area, the scales fell from my eyes: What if I had NICOs? I had never considered the possibility until then. We took a 3-D X-ray to make a conventional dentistry diagnosis and lo and behold: Where the wisdom teeth once sat, there were three huge osteolyses—areas with visible, severe bone degradation. After further testing we eventually found four huge NICOs. We then booked me in for surgery.

NICO is actually an abbreviation for "neuralgia-inducing cavitational osteonecrosis" and comes from the field of pathology.[4] The term isn't strictly accurate, because the eroded bone structure can only be seen on a 3-D X-ray. Ultimately, the term refers to chronically inflamed areas in the jaw. They can appear anywhere where a tooth has been removed. Typically, they occur where wisdom teeth grow, as these are the areas where the most teeth are taken out. But NICOs

## The Madness of Wisdom Tooth Operations

I well remember the first wisdom tooth removal I carried out. My boss at the time had thrown me in at the deep end. The patient was a young girl accompanied by her mother. My boss told me to get started and he would be with me in a moment. But he didn't return for ages. After one hour, I had removed two teeth in tiny steps. Finally my boss returned and removed the remaining two teeth in ten minutes. When the girl came back the next day for a checkup, the side I had worked on was fine, while the other side was badly swollen. I'm convinced that the more gently an operation is carried out, the fewer complications, the less swelling, and the less subsequent pain arises. There's a saying in dentistry that goes: "The best surgeons make the biggest cuts." I would add to this: "and maximum trauma." In routine practice, however, slow and considerate surgery is rarely possible due to costs and time pressure. It's much more common to remove all teeth as quickly as possible in just one step.

can occur following the extraction of any tooth. Strictly speaking, a NICO is therefore not really a disease, but the consequence of disease if the wound does not heal optimally following the removal of a tooth.

If a tooth is removed from the periodontium, it leaves behind a big, gaping wound. A wound in normal tissue, such as the arm or the leg, usually heals without any issues within ten days. But a wound in the bone tissue heals very differently. It's not only the healing process, but in fact the buildup of bone that requires a lot of support from the body. Ironically, wisdom teeth operations are usually required at a time when physical health is not a top priority: in the teens. The average patient is fifteen to twenty years of age when they have their wisdom teeth removed, which means they don't always eat the healthiest food and often like to party, drink alcohol, or smoke. At least 50 percent of patients have complications or serious issues following a wisdom tooth removal. They suffer from hellish pains or have to come back for follow-up treatment.

If our bodies are not in a position to rebuild the bone structure and new tissue after the removal of a tooth, the wound left behind after extraction is merely superficially closed. The body is then able to form a thin, superficial layer of bone over the area of the wound. It eventually feels as though the wound has fully healed. On the inside, however, there is no real bone, but often a fatty, degenerate mass. Nowadays I carry out NICO operations almost on a daily basis. I often see yellow, mushy, degenerate bones where solid, white, cancellous bone should be. There is often part of the osteonecrosis hanging on the underside of the bone flap. I like to describe this part as a pizza, because it looks like a slice of pizza topped with tomato sauce and melted cheese. It can easily be detached from the bone wall and removed by hand with the help of fine surgical tools. Once the wound is perfectly cleaned, it can be disinfected with ozone before an endogenous matrix is applied (see "A Guide to Treating NICOs" on page 124).

When the removed tissue is examined, there are often metals, pesticides, and other environmental toxins present, as well as fungi, viruses, and bacteria inside it.[5]

We now know this thanks above all to holistic dentist Dr. Johann Lechner, who carried out a great many studies on the subject and is regarded as a pioneer in the field. Due to the change in metabolism, certain bacteria seem to make themselves particularly at home in these areas.

NICOs can cause horrible symptoms, because the trigeminal nerve often lies in the middle of the inflamed area. The trigeminal nerve is one of the twelve cranial nerves in the body with a direct connection to the brain. Amazingly, it occupies 50 percent of the space allocated to all the cranial nerves put together. If this nerve is embedded in a primary center of inflammation and therefore becomes inflamed itself, the body suffers a stress response on the one hand; on the other hand the event can cause severe neuralgia (chronic pain). An

## The Visibility of NICOs

One of the reasons why NICOs remained undiscovered for so long is that they are often difficult to find. Generally speaking, they are difficult to spot on an X-ray. They can be found earlier using digital volume tomography, or DVT, but doctors have to be trained to find them in this way. They can also be found radiologically, using computed tomography (CT) scans or bone density measurement technology (the Hounsfield scale), which show whether the bone in the area is fatty.

unfortunate scenario that commonly occurs is patients experiencing unexplained pain that they are not able to localize. Sometimes they feel pain in one tooth, then it moves to another. This is mainly because the trigeminal nerve in the jaw has branches that spread widely in many different directions.

Some people suffer the worst pain imaginable as a result of NICOs, but for a long time nobody can help them. They often seek help from their own doctor or from other doctors to no avail. Many receive one or more—unnecessary—root canal treatments in the affected area. Some are dismissed as crazy. This is a disastrous situation and a consequence of the fact that most dentists are unfamiliar with NICOs. This is because NICOs are not yet taught at universities, and what is not taught at universities simply does not exist for most doctors.

But NICOs can also be a silent problem that goes completely unnoticed, which means they pose the same risks as a tooth that becomes infected after root treatment. They provide the perfect hideout for anaerobic bacteria and are a common cause for diseases that cause inflammation. Typically, patients suffering from NICOs experience chronic fatigue due to the constant activation of the stress axis as a result of the continuous production of cortisol, adrenaline, and noradrenaline. The body essentially ends up burned out. Bowel problems are also common (due to the relationship with the small intestine meridian—see the tooth-organ relationship chart, figure 2.7), as are heart rhythm disturbances and restlessness (due to cortisol), and skin and joint problems. Ultimately, any symptoms can arise when the body is under chronic stress.

Every day I come across people who are suddenly practically cured once NICOs are surgically removed and cared for, and I have also experienced tremendous and rapid relief myself. During my own operation, I even noticed in the operating theater that my back pain had disappeared, and I had to laugh because I could hardly believe it. The next day, the inner restlessness had disappeared, and a week after the operation, my skin looked like that of a Dr. Hauschka model.

## Case Study: Why Do Wisdom Teeth Have to Be Removed at All?

Why don't our wisdom teeth fit properly in our jaws? We've now simply come to terms with the fact that this is the case. But is it normal? If we look at the teeth of humans that lived before us, they were well developed and straight, and wisdom teeth had plenty of room. But by the twentieth century, wisdom teeth removal has become one of the most common surgical procedures in the Western world.[6] Jaw malformation is a much more recent phenomenon. This is often attributed to the fact that the human brain became very large at some point in history, while the jaw started to get smaller. It could have also been the other way around, but there is no way of knowing. In any case, we know that monkeys chew for up to seventeen hours a day. Now that humans cook their food, they chew a lot less. It seems logical that their jaws would shrink. But at some point, this change progressed so rapidly that it could no longer be explained by natural evolution. The epidemic of malpositioned teeth might in fact be a sign that our jaws are not developing properly because we do not feed ourselves properly.[7] The issue of our mouths becoming more and more tightly packed has become worse since we started to grind, refine, and pre-package food. This was another issue Weston Price looked at. Wherever he found populations of people that still ate natural foods, he also found perfect jaws and physiques. They had straight teeth, straight backs, no scoliosis (curvature of the spine), and generally speaking all of their teeth fit into their mouths. Things were very different for people who already had access to white flour and sugar. Price came to the conclusion—with which I also agree—that the lack of space in our mouths is actually a nutrition problem resulting from (micro)nutrient deficiency.

## Teeth and Toxicology

Symptoms usually appear first on the face, with cramps contorting the mouth. Some people can barely open their mouths and have difficulty swallowing. Later on, whole muscle groups in the torso can sometimes cramp so badly that vertebrae in the spine break. I'm talking about tetanus. Tetanus is an infection, yet none of these horrible symptoms are directly caused by bacteria; they are caused by toxins.

Just like humans, microorganisms have a metabolism. They consume and excrete. Sometimes, as is the case with tetanus, it isn't the bacteria themselves that the human organism reacts to, but their metabolites: bacterial toxins. Toxins emanating from infected teeth or NICOs are not only an immunological burden on our immune systems, but also a toxicological one. The bacteria often found in teeth after root canal treatments and in NICOs produce hydrogen sulfide compounds such as thioethers and mercaptans. The tissue remnants left in root canals that have not been completely cleared are also a problem. Our body always tries to break down dead tissue, creating substances that sound incompatible from their names alone: cadaverine and putrescine. Put simply, these are decomposition products, and their presence is very typical in teeth that are inflamed or have undergone root canal treatments.

Toxins can cause other types of strain on the body aside from inflammation. There is no case as violent and acute as the toxins produced by tetanus bacteria. They do not attack particularly quickly or violently; rather they poison the body with a slow, low dose of toxins that disturb the function of another important part of our body: enzymes.

**Enzyme Blockers and Energy Thieves**

Biologists also refer to enzymes as catalysts because there's one thing they can do particularly well: change one substance into another. They do this, for example, by splitting substances up to make them usable for the body. One enzyme that is well known for its ability to break down lactose is lactase. Many adults are not able to produce this enzyme and therefore can't digest dairy particularly well, which is why they soon experience problems if they treat themselves to a rich ice cream. It's possible to live with lactose intolerance by simply avoiding dairy products. But this shows how great an effect the failure of a single enzyme can have on the body.

There are countless enzymes in the body that are involved in a wide variety of tasks: Many work closely with the smallest living units in our bodies, the cells, helping with cell division, repair, and DNA damage. If we could zoom in on these tiny building blocks that we are made up of, we would be able to see what are known as the mitochondria. These are sometimes referred to as the "power plants" of the cells because they provide energy for our bodies. Mitochondria are tiny machines that never stop for as long as we live. Some cells in our bodies have more mitochondria than others because they need more energy than others, such as our muscles. But to be able to produce any energy at all, mitochondria have to work very closely with enzymes. Toxins that emanate from inflammatory processes in the mouth are particularly nasty because they dock onto enzymes, thereby blocking them and preventing them from performing their task properly. This then slows down cell division, for example, making us age faster. These toxins can also affect the work that enzymes carry out in the mitochondria. If enzymes are no longer working properly, the power plants for our cells are affected. Thousands of cogs are constantly interlocking in our organism to make it run. If one fails, this affects all the others.

If our energy power plants no longer function properly, this logically becomes noticeable, mainly because the body has less energy available. When our mitochondria are not able to function properly, experts call this secondary mitochondriopathy. In certain circumstances people are born with mitochondriopathy, but more often than not they acquire it as a result of environmental (epigenetic) factors, which often include toxins and other poisonous substances. Internal process are slowed down in people with secondary mitochondriopathy, leading them to feel the same way: suffocated. All metabolic processes are restricted, which in turn has an effect on all of the body's important systems, such as the cardiovascular, hormone, and immune systems. Scientists are currently researching mitochondriopathy rather diligently, as it is becoming more and more obvious that it triggers and enhances some of the chronic diseases that are so common today.

In addition to chronic inflammation centers, there is another significant source of toxins in our mouths: heavy metals.

## Metals in the Mouth? Never the Right Solution

For the last fifty years, it has been standard practice to fill teeth with metal. After all, dentistry was understood to be a handicraft first and foremost, which is why people put their faith in materials that promised durability and easy processing above all. Whether or not the body is able to handle these materials has rarely come into question up until now.

Amalgam and gold alloy are all still used, mainly because health insurance companies pay for them. Unfortunately, it isn't the overall health of the patient that is the most important for these companies, but that the materials used are "sufficient and appropriate"—in other words, as cheap as possible—as stated in paragraph 28, section 2 of the fifth German social security statute book. Of course, each person is free to choose the material they want, but they then have to pay the remaining costs themselves. Health insurance policies only cover costs that would be incurred for the cheapest option, or, in their words, "economic and necessary." The cheapest option is unfortunately still amalgam. Exceptions can be made for the more visible front teeth. Health insurance pays for slightly better-quality, light-colored composite fillings in this case. Since July 2018 dentists are no longer allowed to use amalgam in adolescents, pregnant women, or nursing mothers.

Most dentists don't have a problem with this, because they learn at school that amalgam works well and has been used for a long time in

## Is Composite Really That Much Better?

*Composite* is the term used to describe any mixture made of plastic and ceramic. These mixtures contain many substances that may cause allergies. Composite is not a particularly ideal material for fillings, although it is a hundred times less toxic than amalgam. Problematic substances in composite include bisphenol glycidyl methacrylate (BisGMA), urethane dimethacrylate (UDMA), "thinners"—co-monomers such as hydroxyethyl methacrylate (HEMA) and triethylene glycol dimethacrylate (TEGDME)—as well as plasticizers such as bisphenol A.[8] Some mixtures contain more of these substances than others. Patients who are sensitive to these should ask their dentists about the composition, and if necessary, have the respective materials tested in an immunological laboratory examination (preliminary testing).

these procedures. It just shouldn't be used for pregnant women and children. Oh, and one more thing: If an amalgam filling has to be taken out, it should be thrown away in the hazardous waste bin.

I have never understood how it can be okay to use amalgam in patients if this is the case. Incidentally, this doesn't happen everywhere. In many countries amalgam has been completely banned as a dental material. Although dentists incorporate most foreign substances into the body immediately after they come from the orthopedist, they don't learn very much about their effects and compatibility. As a dentist, if you want to find out what materials will work with the human body, you have to look to other disciplines. Biochemists know very well, for example, what effect low dosages and the chronic toxicity of metals have on the human organism.

Metal ions are positively charged and, like toxins, they like to bind with enzymes. Metal ions, however, are even more obtrusive—they

## A Dangerous Mishmash

Virtually every metal is alien to our immune system and can therefore trigger an allergy. Patients rarely suspect that they might have introduced into their mouths metals that they are allergic to. Generally speaking fillings use not one but several metals to ensure the desired strength and durability. Gold, platinum, copper, cobalt, iron, and chromium are most common. But patients are not usually told what exactly is in a filling or inlay. This is because, according to the German Medicinal Products Act, only components that constitute over 1 percent of any given material have to be listed. Nickel, for example, can often be found in old amalgam fillings—and many people are allergic to nickel. Today mixtures should all be nickel-free.

Allergic reactions do not depend on the amount or number of allergens in the body, because the body reacts to allergens regardless of the quantity present. It doesn't necessarily take a lot of metal crowns and inlays to spark a reaction. Some people begin to make antibodies when even the smallest amounts of metal are present. This often leads to a low-dose activation of the immune system. Sometimes patients only suffer from minimal localized gum bleeding, while others feel the immune response every day in the form of body aches, slightly elevated temperature, or ongoing sickness and exhaustion. We can assume from this kind of reaction that the body requires a lot of energy to deal with chronic, low-level activation of the immune system. In the case of type IV allergies, the mouth should always be the first port of call for patients and doctors alike. Often the cause of the allergy is quite literally right in front of their noses.

also bind with red blood cells, proteins, and the membranes of nerve cells, as well as interfering with the work of immune messengers and neurotransmitters. When such important areas and communication pathways in our bodies are disrupted or blocked, this can essentially lead to any type of disease: allergies, autoimmune diseases, dementia, hormone disruption, and even diseases of the gut. That's not to say that amalgam is to blame for everything; rather, the heavy metals it contains can play a significant role in a number of diseases.

What exactly is amalgam? *Amalgam* is the generic term for all metal mixtures containing mercury, which makes it a so-called alloy (in Arabic: "melting ointment"). The mercury component of amalgam is always at least 50 percent, while other metals are mixed in varying amounts, meaning there are many different types of amalgam that all differ significantly in their properties. People with multiple amalgam fillings therefore have several different alloys in their teeth.

One of the reasons why amalgam is still used in dentistry is the argument that the materials are firmly bound in the filling once they have been mixed and therefore cannot cause any harm to the patient at all. Unfortunately this isn't true. A small amount of mercury vapor is released daily through everyday processes such as chewing, grinding, brushing teeth, and drinking hot or cold drinks. These amounts may be in the microgram range, but where mercury is concerned, even this can be enough to produce a toxic effect. It has been proven that even one molecule of mercury can destroy nerve cells. Mercury is considered to be the most toxic nonradioactive element, surpassing all other known elements including lead, cadmium, and arsenic—sometimes by far. In tests carried out on animals, a pathological change in the brain could be detected after just fourteen days of wear.[9] If approximately two to three micrograms of mercury vapor is released from a filling per day, this is classed as low-dose, chronic poisoning. On average amalgam fillings last for twenty years. In several studies roughly a two- to fivefold increase of mercury was observed in the blood and urine of living amalgam carriers. In tests on deceased patients, two to twelve times this amount was found in body tissues. There are other sources from which we ingest mercury, such as fish. But amalgam is still the main source of mercury in the body.

## Lurking in the Depths of Our Body Fat

Mercury is fat-soluble, which is why our body stores it mainly in connective or fatty tissue. It's especially problematic for people who have a low body fat percentage or are very athletic; in fact, holding on to a few extra pounds may be worth the price, because if the body doesn't have sufficient fat deposits available, toxins are more often than not deposited in the nerve tissue or in the brain (given that the brain consists mainly of fat), which is more dangerous. Mercury can also get into the placenta. The amount of mercury found in breast milk and in amniotic fluids correlates exactly to the quantity of amalgam fillings in the mother's mouth. Women who want to have children would do best to have their amalgam fillings removed before a planned pregnancy—of course while taking maximum precautions (see "Removal of Metals" on page 120).

## Deadly Gases

Many people only start experiencing problems once amalgam has been removed. But this is no reason to leave amalgam in the body. Rather, it demonstrates the consequences of amalgam fillings being removed far too often without sufficient protective measures, which can have a fatal impact on the patient's health, as well as the health of the practitioner. One of mercury's properties is quick vaporization, which means it turns into gas and rises into the air. This gas is tasteless and odorless so you don't notice when you come into contact with it. But it can penetrate body tissue such as skin, connective tissue, muscles and even bones. It can also easily pass through the blood-brain barrier. There is no barrier in the body strong enough to protect us from mercury. This is something our dentists have to do, which is expensive (see "Removal of Metals" on page 120). This is why many doctors advise leaving mercury where it is. My advice is the opposite; if health, rather than chewing capacity, is the focus, amalgam should be removed in all cases to end this ongoing low-dosage poisoning of the body. Maximum protection measures should be taken, however, to ensure that no more mercury is absorbed than would normally happen on a daily basis.

## Every Body Reacts Differently

Sensitivity to toxic substances in the mouth varies from person to person. Every organism has its own individual tolerance to substances, depending on how well it can detoxify. Experts also speak of susceptibility, or how sensitive biological organisms are to external influences. Early miners took advantage of the fact that canaries have a much higher susceptibility to methane and carbon monoxide than humans do. A cage with a canary inside was often hung in the poorly ventilated coal seams. The miners knew they were safe for as long as the bird continued to sing. A dead canary was a warning to evacuate immediately. Being sensitive to certain things can be a survival advantage, because it enables some people to notice toxic substances faster than others. But in today's world, where we are exposed to many harmful influences, it can be a curse. Being able to do things better than another person, however, is not just coincidence or the result of good genes. It also has a lot to do with how we live and feed ourselves. Today we like to say that things depend on lifestyle factors. Because how we shape our lives and how we feed ourselves has a big impact on how well we can detoxify. This process is also known as biotransformation and takes place in the liver. Today we often hear the term *detox*, which is a cooler way of saying *detoxification*—the removal of poison from the body. It makes no difference to the liver whether a substance is poisonous or not. The liver simply transforms substances so that they can be excreted through the intestines, kidneys, or skin. This process, which I refer to as the body's sanitary service, is highly laborious and costly to the body. In this case the currency is not money but nutrients and micronutrients, in particular protein and its smaller components: amino acids. Our bodies must always be able to dispose of the substances we consume in our diets and medicines, as well as environmental toxins. The ability to detoxify is of utmost importance to our health.

## Case Study: Methylation

Heavy metals and other toxins are rendered water-soluble through the process of methylation and can be eliminated without causing too much damage. The methylation process is disrupted in many people as a result of an enzyme defect known as the MTHFR defect. How effectively a person is able to methylate depends on how well equipped they are with elemental nutrients—in particular, folic acid in its bioactive form, vitamin $B_{12}$, vitamin $B_6$, betaine, magnesium, and protein. Foods that are particularly rich in these substances include green leafy vegetables, red meat (beef, lamb, and so on), eggs, salmon, chicken, and almonds. Pizza, pasta, bread, and biscuits do not contain these (and are also often mixed with synthetic folic acid, which can block the methylation function). What we eat therefore has a significant impact on our ability to detoxify. Moodiness, aggression, headaches, swollen hands, flatulence, tension, so-called brain fog, food intolerances, and concentration problems are just a some of the issues that can arise as a result of a detoxification problem.

Surprisingly, it's the poisons themselves that prevent the organism from being able to detoxify. In other words, toxins such as heavy metals also impede the crucial process of detoxification by blocking important detoxification enzymes and receptors. Over time more and more toxic substances flood the body, making it more and more difficult for the body to get rid of all of them. Almost all the chronically ill patients I treat in my practice have difficulty detoxifying and suffer from one or more of the detoxification mutations known as SNPs (pronounced *snips*—single nucleotide polymorphisms). In addition to the problem of methylation, there are nearly infinite other very specific gene mutations. It would be impossible to count every one of them, but some important ones to note include the COMT gene mutation (catechol-O-methyltransferase), which leads to methylation issues; adrenaline and noradrenaline in particular are not able to break down well or quickly enough. That is to say, the process makes it

## Flushing Valuable Substances Down the Toilet

*HPU* is the abbreviation for a metabolic disease known as hemopyrrollactamuria. People—predominantly women—who are affected by HPU excrete unphysiologically high amounts of vitamin $B_6$, zinc, and sometimes manganese in their urine on a daily basis. This is disastrous because our body desperately needs these micronutrients for detoxification. Unfortunately, these individuals often suffer from detoxification disorders. Methylation ability is also often severely limited. HPU is often genetically determined but it can also be triggered by heavy metal pollution (generally toxins and/or microorganisms). Those affected often feel exhausted, are not resistant to illness, and frequently suffer from allergies and irritable bowel syndrome. In these cases, patients have no option but to take supplements on a long-term basis. This kind of therapy is known as a genetic bypass. It is, however, of utmost importance to optimize nutrition, avoid all harmful influences, and remove or treat factors that can actively disrupt the body's processes, such as metals, infected root canal treatments, and NICOs. This way, the body does not need as many micronutrients.

difficult for the body to be able to "come down" after being activated. These patients generally have difficulty breaking down anesthetic, which usually contains an adrenaline derivative.

In the first step, known as the phase 1 conversion reaction, the respective substance (say, caffeine) is converted into a reactive intermediate product. This process requires many vitamins and micronutrients, in particular B vitamins and, as always, a lot of amino acids. The waste products are tied up in a plastic bag and put outside the front door, so to speak. During the second step, the phase 2 conjugation reaction, the intermediate product is rendered water-soluble so it can be excreted via the liver or the gut. This phase 2 reaction can be described as rubbish collection—picking up the trash bags and transporting them away. But this incredibly important process is not effective in many people—in particular chronically ill patients, who simply become more and more "toxic." It isn't the SNPs that need to be treated in these cases, but the people. And the best form of treatment is a change in diet. Nutrition and micronutrients play a significant role in treating SNPs. Amino acids—the smallest components of proteins and B vitamins—are particularly important. As soon as the source of toxins is removed from the oral cavity (metals, dead teeth, and NICOs) and the detoxification process is supplemented with extra nutrients, patients begin to see massive improvements.

## A Rotten Mix

The only thing worse than having metal in the mouth is having a mixture of metals in the mouth. If, for example, a person has processed gold and amalgam in their teeth, a phenomenon known as the battery effect or galvanic element occurs. This is due to the simple fact that electricity flows between two different metals when placed in a conductive fluid. Saliva, with its high mineral content, is one such fluid. Aside from the constant flow of electricity this causes, metal corrodes faster in such conditions, thereby releasing more metal ions. The metal therefore becomes even more toxic, and its allergy potential increases. Amalgam and gold are often found together in the mouth, even if dentists are taught at school not to put them together. Often a buildup of gold can be found on a titanium implant. Gold and titanium are far apart in the electrochemical series, which means they have a particularly high voltage potential: Cases of up to three and a half volts have been measured. Although we learn during our studies never to use different metals in dentistry procedures, it happens quite often in practice because dentists usually treat patients tooth by tooth, without looking at the entirety of the work carried out in the mouth. But even if all the teeth in a person's mouth were treated with only one kind of metal, the battery effect could still take place, because alloys (made in laboratories) are often created at different times and therefore have different proportions of added metals.

## Gold

Gold was once the standard material used in dentistry, because it was considered a neutral, durable material. We now know better. In an immunotoxological evaluation carried out by means of LTT tests (lymphocyte transformation testing for the determination of type IV immune reaction to metals) on metals in 1,120 patients, gold came just after nickel, inorganic mercury, and cadmium: fourth place in a list of the most common allergies. (See figure 2.6.)[10]

Previously, gold alloys were used directly after the removal of amalgam as the preferred material for crowns and partial crowns. The problem here is that the tooth is not given the opportunity to detoxify

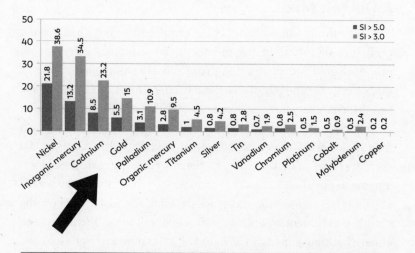

**Figure 2.6.** Alarming statistics on the use of gold. These are the results of lymphocyte transformation testing (LTT) in 1,120 patients. Nickel is at the top of the list of the most common metals found in fillings, closely followed by inorganic mercury. Gold and palladium come in just after cadmium. The stimulation index (SI) shows how many people had a more severe immune reaction (SI > 5) compared with a less extreme but still significant one (SI > 3). Data from Bieger laboratory in Munich.

## First Things First

Before starting an active detox, or even follow-up therapy with an environmental or alternative medicine practitioner, the source of the toxin (the amalgam filling, gold/metal crown, tooth with root canal treatment, or NICO) must be removed. This is where the most disastrous mistakes are often made, which can have serious consequences. Dr. Dietrich Klinghart and Dr. Joachim Mutter are, in my opinion, two of the most knowledgeable and experienced therapists in the field of integrative medicine, and in particular in the removal of heavy metals. They both agree on one thing in particular: The first priority should be to remove the source.

from the remaining heavy metal ions. Rather, any mercury residues remain in the tooth because of the new gold in the tooth, since the two metals have a high affinity for each other. Often amalgam is left in the tooth and a new layer of gold is simply added on top of it, something I see frighteningly often—in around 50 percent of cases—of all the metal crowns I remove.

### Titanium

Titanium is the metal most commonly used in implants. It's used in 99 percent of cases. Titanium is considered to be high-quality, durable, and very resistant. Many patients have a high tolerance for titanium, but according to Volker von Baehr from the Berlin Potsdam Institute for Medical Diagnostics, increasing numbers of people are sensitive to titanium (di)oxide—currently 15 to 20 percent. This is not only because so many people have titanium implants in their mouths, but because titanium dioxide is used frequently in all sorts of everyday items. As a white dye (E171), it's a component of toothpaste, sun cream, cosmetics, and nutritional supplements. It can also be found in paints, varnishes, and other types of dye. Frequent contact can cause a person's immune system to become sensitized to titanium and no longer tolerate it. This can lead to all kinds of symptoms associated with everything from allergies to autoimmune diseases.[11]

### Peri-Implantitis

Sometimes titanium implants simply do not work. They heal badly or cause a nasty inflammation around themselves until eventually the patient loses the implant completely. This is known as peri-implantitis. Implants require special care and there are certain risk factors, such as smoking or a generally poor state of health, that prevent the implant from lasting very long. But sometimes the area can flare up even if there are no—or few—risk factors. Often in these cases, the cause is the metal itself. Scientists know that when a titanium implant is screwed in, oxide particles detach from the surface and penetrate the tissue. In one animal study, titanium oxide particles were even found in regional lymph nodes.[12] The immune system then responds by releasing immunocytokines after the tissue macrophages have eaten the particles. This results in local inflammation, which then turns into chronic inflammation because the implant remains in the body rather than being removed. Locally, this can lead to increased osteoclast activity, which results in increased bone resorption. But this type of chronic inflammation can also lead to serious systemic problems.

## Metals and Inflammation: A Deadly Combination

On August 14, 1996, American chemistry professor Karen Wetterhahn had a fatal accident in her laboratory while studying the toxicity of metals. During one experiment, a small amount of dimethylmercury ran onto her hand and burned through her glove onto her skin. A few months later, Wetterhahn began to suffer from dizziness and headaches, before falling into a coma and later dying from acute mercury poisoning. The concentration of mercury in her blood was eighty times the toxic threshold.

## Electrosensitivity

Those with metals in their mouths are also susceptible to problems caused by something called electro-smog. The electronic networks around us are becoming increasingly complex thanks to Wi-Fi and cell phones. Metals in the body act as little antennae that can completely disrupt the action potential of the cells. This leads to the buildup of electric fields, which can disrupt the nervous system. The standard absorption rate of electromagnetic fields can increase four hundred to seven hundred times from cell phone use alone (both for calling and sending/receiving SMS) in combination with metals in the mouth.[13] Patients with electrosensitivities in particular should therefore not have any metals in their mouths. Electrosensitivity can cause a lack of concentration, memory loss, and insomnia, as well as nonspecific symptoms such as stinging or pressure in the chest area, inexplicable irregular heartbeat, and tinnitus.

Metals are toxic enough to our organisms. But combined with bacterial toxins, their toxicity increases drastically again. Dimethylmercury, which caused Karen Wetterhahn's death, can also be produced in low concentrations in the body when heavy metals and bacterial metabolic products such as mercaptans and thioethers come into contact and bind with one another. This fatal combination can be found, for example, when root-canal-treated teeth and teeth filled with amalgam are adjacent. I describe the combination of an amalgam filling and a tooth that has undergone root canal treatment as a time bomb, because it can create super toxins such as dimethylmercury, which is completely lipophilic. This means that it can pass through our cell membranes unhindered, enter the cell nucleus, and nest there. The only way of getting rid of these substances is for the cell to die, which fortunately happens naturally as every cell has an expiration date. As always, the dose is what makes the substance toxic. If a person is allergic to a substance, however, the dose is irrelevant because the immune system will react to even the tiniest amounts. Inflammation and toxins in the mouth not only put enormous strain on our immune system, but also affect the nervous system.

## Teeth and the Nervous System

If a patient goes to their orthopedist with complaints about a pain in their right shoulder, hopefully the orthopedist will think to look not only at the right shoulder itself, but also the patient's liver and gallbladder. The right shoulder is located next to the right ear, the gallbladder in the upper abdomen. Why should an orthopedist connect the two? The simple answer is that everything in our body is connected via the nervous system. Every last part of us is alive and continually receives stimuli, which are passed on through a gigantic, superfast data network. This enables us to absorb, process, and respond to everything that happens around us in an instant. But our nervous system is nowhere near as straightforward as we might imagine. There's no specific nerve for the left little finger, for example, that feeds it information. Rather, a nerve is usually responsible for entire composite systems, also known by scientists as segments. This is mainly due to the way in which humans develop at the beginning of their lives. From the small cluster of cells we begin our lives as, our limbs form; they grow in length before, finally, nerve pathways begin to emerge. We begin our lives as a sort of bean, but then we develop as the original tissues shift and move away from one another, a bit like the earth's tectonic plates. Although Australia and Europe are far away from each other, they were once part of the same landmass. The common source does not suddenly cease to exist. The same applies to our bodies, which is why organs that are located far away from each other are sometimes on the same meridian. If a part of the body is paired with a section of skin, this is known as a dermatome, or a myotome if it's paired with muscles.

So when a person asks, "Why do I have constant shoulder pain?" in reality they may be experiencing pain caused by problems in the organ the shoulder is paired with (its dermatome). Neural therapy takes advantage of this phenomenon and often treats organs via their corresponding segments.

When there is a problem rooted in the mouth, sometimes we feel it in the neck area rather than the mouth itself. If someone tells me they have neck problems, I always suspect that their teeth are to blame. This is because the myotome for mouth issues are segments CI to CIV, an area that roughly corresponds to the area between the shoulder and skull. Almost all of my patients experience a noticeable change in the flexibility of their cervical spine following successful rehabilitation treatment in the mouth.

The nerves can be stimulated in both directions, which is why acupressure and acupuncture tend to be effective and why a massage can be incredibly beneficial. It is possible to send impulses to underlying connective tissues via certain areas of skin. In traditional Chinese medicine nerve connections have played an important role for over four thousand years. These pathways are known as meridians and show acupuncturists the connections between areas of skin and remote regions of the body, as well as between individual teeth and organ units.

I had just begun to study this theory when I experienced an impressive demonstration of how much tooth-organ relationships can affect a person's life. During my assistantship a young man ended up on my dentist's chair. He was twenty-four and had been doing professional judo for four years. He was physically and athletically at his peak, until he began experiencing mysterious symptoms. Each night, at a specific time, he started to feel so sick he had to vomit. Of course, he went to see a doctor. And then another, and then another, but none of the doctors could pinpoint the problem. He didn't have an acute infection, a gastric ulcer, or an allergy. There didn't seem to be any physical cause for his suffering. He came to me by accident because he needed dental treatment. By this time, he had already been labeled psychosomatic. To see him, you wouldn't have thought he was an athlete. He was pale, weak, and clearly run-down from the last few

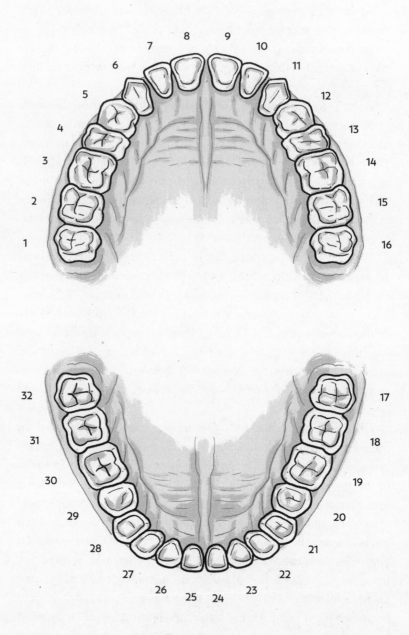

**Figure 2.7.** The tooth-organ relationship chart.

**1**: Inner ear, shoulder, elbow, right side of heart, small intestine, allergies, posterior pituitary gland, CNS, psyche

**2**: Jaw, front of knee, pancreas, right side of stomach, parathyroid, thyroid, right mammary gland

**3**: Jaw, front of knee, pancreas, right side of stomach, thyroid, right mammary gland

**4**: Shoulder, elbow, hand radial, foot, big toe, lung, large intestine, thymus

**5**: Shoulder, elbows, hand radial, foot, big toe, lung, large intestine, thymus, posterior pituitary

**6**: Back of knee, hip, foot, gallbladder, posterior pituitary, right side of liver

**7** and **8**: Back of knee, coccyx, right kidney, right side of bladder, urogenital area, epiphyses, back issues, headaches

**9** and **10**: Back of knee, coccyx, hip, foot, left kidney, left side of bladder, urogenital area, epiphyses, back issues, headaches

**11**: Hip, left side of liver, left bile duct, posterior pituitary gland

**12**: Shoulder, elbow, hand radial, foot, big toe, lung, large intestine, posterior pituitary gland

**13**: Shoulder, elbow, hand radial, foot, big toe, lung, large intestine, posterior pituitary gland, thymus

**14**: Jaw, front of knee, spleen, left side of stomach, left mammary gland

**15**: Jaw, front of knee, spleen, left side of stomach, parathyroid, left mammary gland

**16**: Shoulder, elbow, hand ulnar, foot, plantar, toes, small intestine, allergies, CNS, psyche

**17**: Energy balance, peripheral nerves, left side of heart, circulation, small intestine, allergies, hand ulnar, foot plantar, toes, ear, retina

**18**: Arteries, left lung, left side of large intestine, shoulder, elbow, hand radial, foot, big toe, ethmoidal cells, nose, sense of smell

**19**: Veins, left lung, left side of large intestine, shoulder, elbow, hand radial, foot, big toe, ethmoidal cells, nose, sense of smell

**20**: Left mammary gland, lymph vessel, spleen, front of knee, jaw, maxillary sinus, tongue, sense of taste

**21**: Left mammary gland, gonad, left side of stomach, front of knee, jaw, maxillary sinus, tongue, sense of taste

**22**: Gonad, left side of liver, bile ducts, hip, eye, eyesight

**23** and **24**: Adrenal gland, left kidney, left side of bladder, urogenital area, back of knee, coccyx, hip, foot, frontal sinus, nose, sense of smell

**25** and **26**: Adrenal gland, bladder, urogenital area, back of knee, coccyx, foot, frontal sinus, nose, sense of smell, right kidney

**27**: Gonad, right side of liver, gallbladder, back of knee, foot, eye, eyesight

**28**: Right mammary gland, gonad, pancreas, right side of stomach, pylorus, front of knee, jaw, maxillary sinus, tongue, sense of taste

**29**: Right mammary gland, lymph vessels, pancreas, right side of stomach, pylorus front of knee, jaw, maxillary sinus, tongue, sense of taste

**30** and **31**: Arteries, right lung, right side of large intestine, sacroiliac joint, shoulder, elbow, hand radial, foot, big toe, ethmoidal cells, nose, sense of smell

**32**: Energy balance, peripheral nerves, right side of heart, circulation, small intestine, shoulder, elbow, hand ulnar, foot plantar, toes, ear, retina

years, during which he had fought for his credibility and against an illness that had prevented him from living his normal life. He told me all this as a side note. When he had finished talking, he said: "If you can think of anything, just do it."

I checked him over and found a tooth that had undergone root canal treatment with a giant cyst at its tip. It had had an effect on the colon meridian. I pulled the tooth out and removed the cyst. A few days later, the patient came back to me. After his treatment, he had gone through the night without vomiting for the first time in months. We found out that he had a detoxification problem (SNPs). When I learned that he sometimes earned extra money by soldering computer boards without any protective equipment, I optimized his diet and micronutrient intake, which helped him deal with his detoxification problems. Soon after, he was able to take up his sport at the level he'd competed prior to his health problems.

Today I start each consultation with the tooth-organ relationship chart as standard. In general, the problems my patients describe stem from the corresponding areas on the chart.

## The Autonomic Nervous System

Many people regard the meridian system as alternative mumbo jumbo. But today we know that meridian pathways are simply points of the autonomic nervous system that are particularly easy to stimulate: our internal data motorways.

We send the signals for many of the things our bodies do—to run away, say, or to jump on one leg, or to wink at someone—and our bodies respond accordingly. But there are certain functions they don't let us have a say in—functions they prefer to be in charge of. We can't stop the digestive system, for example, and we're not able to control our salivary glands. The blood flows through our veins whether we like it or not, and even our lungs can breathe by themselves. Our organisms have to constantly adapt to an unpredictable and changing environment and the situations we put them through. We put ourselves into a state of shock by walking out in front of cars or by shoving three chocolate bars into ourselves, one after the other.

## Neural Therapy

Neural therapy procedures can be used to determine which areas to work on to treat which interference fields. Procaine, a local anesthetic, is injected near the affected area—for example, a tooth that has undergone root canal treatment. The patient then observes what changes they experience for one day. It might be that the patient feels more relaxed, that symptoms related to limited mobility suddenly disappear, or that they suddenly start to sweat profusely or giggle like a child because the remote effect of the problem is temporarily relieved. As soon as the effect wears off, the patient's symptoms return. Some patients don't notice anything at all, since they have been out of touch with their bodily sensations for so long. I can see right away when the body switches over to the parasympathetic nervous system from a patient's pupils, which become particularly small.

For our bodies, this means either cooling us down or warming us up. The body shoots adrenaline through our veins so that we can jump out of danger in time and lowers blood sugar levels that have shot through the ceiling after the chocolate bars. We all have our own internal thermostat, which keeps our most important parameters constantly within a certain range. The puppet master behind these magical processes is called our autonomic nervous system. It establishes a constant balance in the body because it has two major counterparts: the sympathetic nervous system and the parasympathetic nervous system.

### The Sympathetic Nervous System

The sympathetic nervous system is the activating part of the autonomic nervous system. It's responsible for what is known as the fight-or-flight response—the reactions we need to either escape from danger or fight it. The sympathetic nervous system is what causes each of the following vital body reactions to be triggered:

1. It tightens our blood vessels to make the heart pump faster.
2. It activates muscles to make us run faster.
3. It boosts our energy and widens our pupils.

It also stops all processes that would be a hindrance to us in this mode. Some examples of these processes include our immune system, ability to concentrate, digestion, and secretion of saliva. Nobody fleeing from a dangerous situation is simultaneously thinking about the theory of relativity or stopping for a bite to eat. When we're in sympathetic mode, everything is switched on. The sympathetic nervous system is therefore a powerful puppet master and can influence every one of our organs.

## The Parasympathetic Nervous System

The parasympathetic nervous system, on the other hand, is the system that helps us to rest and digest. When this system is able to take over, it helps us to calm down, to slow down our heart rate, and to activate the digestive system. Only in this mode are our bodies able to relax, regenerate, and refuel. The digestive system ticks over, the liver detoxifies, the glands increase their secretion rate, and the cardiovascular system shuts down.

Some doctors say that to understand the autonomic nervous system is to understand medicine in general. I don't think that's too much of a stretch—in fact, most illnesses occur when something isn't quite right between the sympathetic and parasympathetic nervous systems. Normally our organism switches harmoniously from one system to the other, much like the yin and yang principle in Chinese medicine. It makes sense and is important that our bodies run at full speed sometimes, if we need to react to a problem. But it's just as important that we are able to recover from this mode.

Unfortunately most of us today live lifestyles that trigger the sympathetic nervous system rather than its more chilled-out counterpart, the parasympathetic nervous system. Noise, deadlines, time pressure,

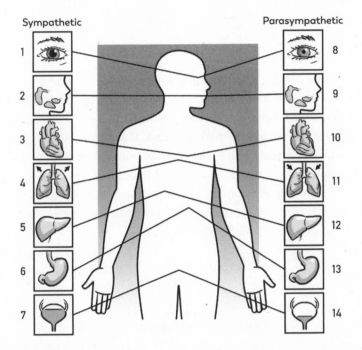

| Sympathetic | Parasympathetic |
|---|---|
| 1 | 8 |
| 2 | 9 |
| 3 | 10 |
| 4 | 11 |
| 5 | 12 |
| 6 | 13 |
| 7 | 14 |

**1**: Widens pupils
**2**: Stops salivation
**3**: Increases heart rate
**4**: Stimulates glucose release
**5**: Stimulates adrenaline and noradrenaline
**6**: Inhibits digestion
**7**: Allows the bladder to relax

**8**: Narrows pupils
**9**: Stimulates salivation
**10**: Decreases heart rate
**11**: Widens lungs
**12**: Stimulates gallbladder
**13**: Stimulates digestion
**14**: Stimulates bladder

**Figure 2.8.** The sympathetic and parasympathetic nervous systems control our entire nervous system.

work and family commitments, worries and fears . . . the sympathetic nervous system is triggered in all situations in which we experience what is commonly described as stress. As a result of this stress, the organs targeted by the sympathetic nervous system are constantly activated instead of just occasionally. Most of us know that we have far too much stress in our lives. But we often overlook the fact that stress doesn't always come from external factors. Fighting infections

## Do Animals Get Stressed?

Fight-or-flight situations trigger the same reactions in humans and animals. But animals have a clear advantage over us: They can handle stress better than we do. Their trick is that they are able to make vitamin C themselves. Vitamin C is an anti-stress vitamin that helps us to break down cortisol, adrenaline, and noradrenaline. All mammals can produce vitamin C except humans and, surprisingly, apes and guinea pigs. It is therefore especially important that we get enough vitamin C, particularly in times of stress.

or chronic inflammation, suffering from allergies, dealing with toxins or dysbiosis (an imbalance in the gut flora) are all sources of internal stress for the body. Our mouths can sometimes be the number one trigger of stress in our lives. We might be able to forget about our bosses at the end of the day, but there are certain forms of stress that we can't set aside because they come from inside our bodies.

## Internal Stress Factors

Stress that comes from inside our bodies basically triggers the same reaction as stress from external factors. But the fact that it never relents, regardless of how much we meditate or how many mandalas we color in, is what makes it all the more serious. All sympathetic reactions that are useful in the short term become potential causes for ill health in the long term. Blood pressure rises and remains high, digestion is disrupted, restlessness becomes constant, muscles stay tensed, and the immune system is inhibited. Reactions that help us in the short term in an emergency situation can make us ill in the long term. Our organism no longer switches among its various mechanisms but remains constantly at the extreme end of

## Neuromodulatory Triggers:
## When Stress Comes from the Inside

Any form of stress caused by toxins, sources of inflammation, or foreign bodies is referred to as a neuromodulatory trigger in neural therapy or as an interference field in complementary medicine. These terms refer to areas in the body in which there are constant pathological impulses. In the tooth and jaw area, there are many such triggers. These include heavy metals, material intolerances, chronic gum inflammation, teeth that have undergone root canal treatment and toxins that come from these, as well as areas in the jawbone that have been chronically altered (NICOs). Our bodies are programmed to detect and respond to any disruptive factors, just like our immune systems. While the body's defense system reacts with immunocytokines, the nervous system responds by releasing neurotransmitters and hormones. These are messenger substances that can initiate a domino effect of reactions because the central nervous system or the hormone system react to them.

the spectrum. If the body stays in sympathetic mode constantly or keeps reentering this mode, this can cause any number of symptoms, including gastrointestinal problems, dizziness, palpitations, depression, impulsive behaviors, sleep disorders, susceptibility to infections, teeth grinding, temporomandibular joint problems (which in turn can cause back and muscle problems), difficulty concentrating, and tension.

Each of these symptoms can lead to a variety of other pathological reactions. Cortisol, for example, blocks the thyroid gland, and a blocked thyroid gland changes the hormonal system. A hormone imbalance can in turn cause infertility, among other things.

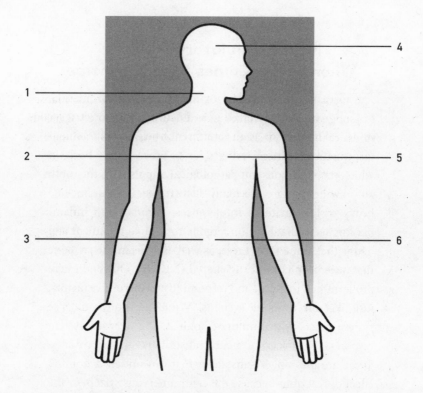

**1**: Tension/headache/spinal problems/exhaustion
**2**: Increased susceptibility to infections
**3**: Increased digestive problems
**4**: Restlessness, neurochemical lapses, serotonin deficiency,
sleep disturbances, concentration difficulties
**5**: Increased risk of heart attack
**6**: Obesity, diabetes, metabolic diseases

**Figure 2.9.** This is the effect that stress has on our organs.

At the same time, our bodies become increasingly exhausted in this situation because they are constantly trying to compensate for the imbalance by producing cortisol (a stress hormone), adrenaline, and noradrenaline. In the long term the little glands that are located on our kidneys can no longer keep up with the work caused by this stress, so they eventually become tired and weak, leading to burnout.

After a period of discomfort and exhaustion, the disruption of bodily functions on a long-term basis can eventually lead to serious illnesses.

The health and well-being of a person essentially depends on how well and how smoothly their immune and nervous systems run. There are many factors in the mouth that cause disturbances or lapses in these supersystems. To understand the influence of dental health on the rest of the body, we first have to understand the immune and nervous systems. Unfortunately we often turn a blind eye to their importance. This is mainly because the mouth is considered to be separate from and outside of the body. Biological dentistry uses the knowledge available to us from other sciences and from functional medicine to treat the body as a whole and to optimize health. Ultimately, biological dentistry is the logical progression from the predominantly handicraft-oriented basic training provided to the dental profession.

# —THREE—

# Teeth and Chronic Disease

When faced with a very big and complex problem, complexity managers like to ask their clients the following question to guide them toward the right approach: "How do you eat an elephant?" The answer is: "One bite at a time."

For years scientists have tackled the human body as if they were facing an overwhelming task—an approach that would be lauded by complexity managers. They break the body down into pieces and look at each in turn. Our immune, nervous, and endocrine systems have been studied and treated separately for a very long time. Traditionally, they are thought of as separate, independent closed-loop systems. But recently it has become increasingly obvious that this is a mistake. It might be easier to understand the body bit by bit, and it might be easier to eat an elephant in this way, too, but unfortunately this method does not give us the answer to a very pressing question of our time: Why do people suffer from chronic diseases?

To find out, researchers are gradually starting to put the body and all of its important parts together again, because it turns out they can be understood much better as a whole. Nerves, hormones, and the immune system do not work independently from one another as we believed for a very long time. Instead there are close correlations among them; they work closely together and mutually influence one another. Neurotransmitters stimulate hormones, which in turn affect the immune system, which in turn affects the organism as a whole. Our bodies do not consist of soloists; our health is a polyphonic orchestra. When everyone relies on everyone else, the overall picture is quickly disrupted when there is a problem with just one participant. If one person hits the wrong note in an orchestra, everything sounds a little off. Similarly, health is something that you have until something disrupts it.

## Are We Getting Sicker or Just Older?

People often mistakenly believe that we are seeing more chronically ill people today because people are getting older. In the past we simply wouldn't have reached an age in which we could get chronically ill in the first place. Of course average life expectancy has increased, but it has also been proven that chronic diseases have simultaneously increased among young people. Type 2 diabetes, for example, is no longer a symptom of old age. It affects increasing numbers of children and adolescents, too. The onset of allergies and autoimmune diseases is also happening earlier in life.

Our modern lifestyle seriously disrupts the most important participants in our organism. Bad nutrition, environmental influences, chronic inflammatory processes, and stress all have an effect on us. The diseases that are most prevalent in our society today do not arise as a result of strokes of fate that come out of the blue; they evolve because participants in charge of orchestrating our health are constantly being knocked out of tune.

Within a century, the most life-threatening diseases have changed drastically. As recently as the turn of the twentieth century, it was mainly acute infectious diseases such as tuberculosis and measles that we had to fear. Today it is mainly noncommunicable, chronic diseases such as diabetes, cardiovascular diseases, allergies, rheumatic diseases, osteoporosis, gastrointestinal diseases, thyroid disorders, and cancers that pose a threat. The number of people suffering from these diseases is increasing so rapidly that chronic diseases have been referred to as the epidemic of the twenty-first century.

As different as the symptoms might be for each of these diseases, generally speaking they all have one common cause: chronic stress, which directly impacts and disrupts all three supersystems.

## A New Outlook

One of the branches of science that is currently coming to maturity is named, rather exotically, psychoneuroimmunology. The reason it has such a long-winded name is that it tackles a number of disciplines as a whole, rather than separately. It takes into account the interaction of the nervous, immune, and hormonal systems in the body, as well as the effects they have on our organs and psyche. These three supersystems not only have a tremendous effect on physical illness, but also significantly affect our emotional well-being. Psychoneuroimmunology provides a new basis for understanding the biology of diseases and uses these findings for diagnostics and therapy. From this point of view, it is also easier to understand why chronically ill patients often suffer not only from one disease, but from several. Those who suffer from rheumatism often have diabetes, and those with diabetes are more likely to suffer from depression. Doctors describe these patients as multimorbid, and refer to this phenomenon as a multisystem disease. It might sound as though these patients are just particularly unlucky, but this doesn't in fact mean that they have multiple diseases at once. The cause is often the same, but because the three supersystems influence one another and affect many different organs, different symptoms appear. Multisystem diseases develop in vicious circles.

As such, stress can cause disease in the gut, which in turn can affect the immune system. Once the immune system is disrupted, all sorts of systemic diseases can arise.

Our current health care system is primarily reactive to these diseases. It can reduce symptoms, but it pays little attention to individual causes. As a result, many people are likely to remain in a state of disease. If a patient visits a doctor because they have high blood pressure, for example, the doctor will most likely prescribe medication, but won't help the person to pinpoint the cause and direct them in the right way to tackle it. Modern medicine is great at treating acute disease, but it has trouble dealing with chronic disease. This often gives the impression that chronic diseases are a destiny that people simply have to resign themselves to. We have learned to regard chronic illness as normal, unalterable, or simply part of the processes of aging and wear. Many people surrender to the idea that they have just become old. And yet we now know that the majority of chronic diseases are acquired as a result of either lifestyle choices, the wrong diet, or chronic stress factors. The triggers are found particularly often in the mouth, which is too frequently overlooked. Teeth can play a role in almost all diseases people commonly suffer from today because they affect our supersystems. Anyone looking for a solution to improve their health should start with their mouth.

## Chronic Fatigue and Susceptibility to Recurring Infections

It's just as bad to be almost sick as it is to actually be sick. It has become a phenomenon of our time to constantly feel just a little bit sick. We feel like we're getting a fever but it never quite breaks out. We feel constantly lethargic without being able to explain why. Many people today are suffering from "nearly" diseases. They can feel that they're not as fit as they once were, that their mood is clouding over or they are coming down with every virus going. They often have a headache or the feeling that they are looking at the world through a fog. Some become forgetful or have difficulty concentrating. Others suffer from constant indigestion or wonder why they have constant joint pain or a tense neck all the time. Although these kinds of "nearly" diseases affect many people, conventional medicine does not take them as seriously as it ought to.

Patients who visit the doctor with these symptoms are either palmed off from one expert to the next or sent on their way with a vague diagnosis. Many people end up reluctantly giving up the search for a cause or relief because the problem simply doesn't seem to have a concrete source. They believe that age must be the culprit for the seemingly endless list of problems they are experiencing. Our medical system is not well equipped to deal with unspecific symptoms that don't fit a particular clinical picture. Sometimes patients' problems are not even recognized as real symptoms. Constant fatigue and loss of energy are often dismissed as normal. Often patients are labeled hypochondriacs—a term handed out all too often when there seems to be "nothing right" with a patient.

But it is so important to take these phenomena and changes seriously. They are important and should be taken as clear signs that there is something fundamentally wrong in the body—a stressor hiding somewhere in the form of chronic inflammation or another issue. When the body sends signals, it always has a reason for doing so, and it's important that we go and search for the cause. If the cause is in the mouth, it's important to have a thorough checkup with an experienced biological dentist to check whether you have cysts, inflamed root tips, NICOs, or gingivitis.

Because the nervous system is connected to many target organs, stress symptoms can crop up in almost any form. The following symptoms are an indication that the body is dealing with a chronic stressor:

- Constant headache and tiredness.
- Neck and body aches.
- A new rash.
- Constantly bloated stomach.
- Sudden decrease in performance in athletes.
- Finding it hard to get out of bed in the morning.
- Constantly feeling like you have a fever.

It is very typical to have a fever that occurs at certain times of the day, for example from eight to ten in the morning, before it disappears again (because the body becomes used to it), only to come back the next day.

From the perspective of functional medicine and biological dentistry, these kinds of symptoms are not just a hint, but evidence

## Why Pain Is Bad Advice

In dentistry it is common to respond only to very clear signals, such as severe pain or unambiguous symptoms, before treating a patient. In the case of chronic illnesses, it is bad advice to wait until something hurts or causes us significant problems before treating it, because by that time it's usually too late. Almost all chronic diseases such as diabetes, hypertension, or cancer develop silently and without pain.

that the nervous system is stressed as a result of chronic inflammation. If the cause is in the mouth, it should be identified and removed; then the rest of the body should be helped to regenerate to prevent the development of a serious disease.

## Heart and Cardiovascular Diseases

Bacteria from the mouth love the heart. It is one of their absolute favorite organs to target when they start to move out of the mouth to colonize the rest of the body. The heart seems to be a kind of locus minoris resistentiae, the medical term for a weakness in the body that favors the development of disease. Today we know that certain bacteria prefer certain tissues, and bacteria from the mouth prefer the tissues found in and around the heart.

A large number of studies have proven that bacteria from the mouth can promote and trigger the development of cardiovascular diseases. The connection was already apparent decades ago when the progress of medicine at the time suffered from setbacks again and again: Physicians had managed to treat diseased and damaged heart valves with artificial replacements. But even if an operation was successful, the heart valve replacement often became inflamed very quickly, and infections were often fatal. While searching for the cause of infection, physicians repeatedly found bacteria that are normally found in the mouth when they examined the heart. But how did they get there?

We now know that this happens as a result of a very simple process. We chew, we brush our teeth, have tartar removed at the dentist's, or simply floss our teeth. The microlesions and breakup of the biofilm that occur as a result always cause a certain number of bacteria to enter the rest of the organism. Physicians refer to this as bacteremia. In terms of oral flora, a healthy environment is one in which there is a mixture of microorganisms. If we are otherwise healthy, a small bout of oral bacteria doesn't pose any problem at all. Bacteria only become problematic when bad bacteria are allowed to take over as the result of a bad tooth replacement, dead teeth, or NICOs. If, in addition to these problems, the immune system is disrupted or a patient has a preexisting heart condition, the combination can be dangerous. A problem that starts off in the mouth suddenly becomes a problem for the entire body.

Today it is well known that bacteria from the mouth can also be involved in all forms of heart disease, and in particular in heart attacks and strokes—long before they actually happen.

The precursor of many cardiovascular diseases is known as arteriosclerosis. Arteriosclerosis affects the blood vessels that supply our heart with oxygen and nutrients. Our blood vessels are not simply tubes that liquids flow through. If we take a closer look at them, we realize that they are very soft, elastic, and flexible, and that they can react to every one of our emotions. If we are agitated, for example, they become narrow to provide the body with more blood as quickly as possible. When we're relaxed, so are our vessels, and the blood flows through them like a calm river. If we treat our bodies badly, our vessels can start to lose their wonderful qualities. Poor nutrition, for example, can lead to deposits building up on the inner walls.

The vessels lose their elasticity as a result, which acts as a trigger for many other diseases. High blood pressure, stroke, heart attack, and heart failure are some of the deadliest diseases in our society. Before, smoking, obesity, and poor nutrition were all risk factors— and undoubtedly remain risk factors today. But it's becoming increasingly clear that inflammation also plays a major role in the development of arteriosclerosis.

## Taking Things to Heart

Dentists take special protective measures for those with preexisting heart conditions. Because the risk of bacterial overgrowth from dental treatment is so great, dentistry guidelines dictate that they can only be carried out on certain patients under antibiotics. This applies particularly to patients who have a greater risk of developing a heart inflammation known as endocarditis. Above all, this applies to those who:

- Have already suffered from endocarditis.
- Have a congenital cyanotic heart defect.
- Have had a heart defect operated on.

But there is something positive to be taken from these guidelines: If it's so obvious that patients with a previous history of disease need antibiotic protection for their hearts because dysbiosis, inflammation, and metals in their mouths are so dangerous, why not protect the heart by eliminating these potential areas of interference in the first place?

Any kind of deposit in the blood vessels provides a playground for bacteria. Sclerotic vessels have been found to contain bacteria from the mouth.[1] Today, however, the influence of chronic inflammation is considered so serious that it can be treated as an independent risk factor for arteriosclerotic vascular disease and is on a level with elevated blood lipid levels, high blood pressure, and obesity. In other words, we may well be slim, drink green smoothies, and ride a bike to work, but for as long as we have untreated inflammation in the mouth or elsewhere in the body, we might as well be smoking a pack of Marlboros a day.

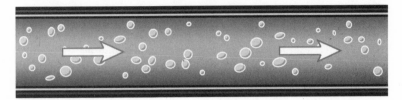

Normal blood flow

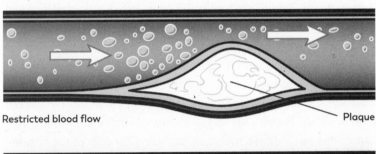

Restricted blood flow                                    Plaque

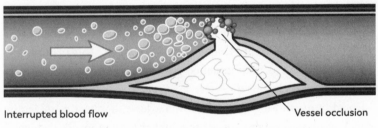

Interrupted blood flow                          Vessel occlusion

Figure 3.1. Bacteria from the mouth can play a role in the narrowing of blood vessels in cases of arteriosclerosis.

You can make a considerable improvement to your health by starting with your mouth. If you incorporate exercise and a healthy diet, you'll also have a happy heart.

## Obesity

There are several interactions between obesity and diseases of the mouth. Some might think that the simple explanation for this is that those who are overweight are more likely to have an unhealthy diet and therefore bad teeth. The truth is it's more complicated than that, but also more interesting. Obesity is considered a risk factor for chronic gingivitis periodontitis. When researchers measure a high body-mass index (BMI), a large waist circumference, and a high waist-hip ratio in a patient, they usually also find periodontitis. It's also true that the higher these values, the more severe the degree of gingivitis.

Why is this? To understand the answer, we need to take a fresh look at our fatty tissues. Body fat can't simply be imagined as a stick of butter or lard. There's not a lot going on in a stick of butter. Body fat, on the other hand, leads such an independent life that scientists go as far as to call it an endocrine organ. Specifically, this means that our extra padding doesn't just hang around doing nothing on our hips. In fact it's quite active and produces a considerable number of bioactive cells and substances. Adipocytes are one example of this type of cell. Adipocytes act both locally and systemically—in the whole body. They can do the same as macrophages, the Pac-Man cells of the immune system. They emit messenger substances. This is why the bodies of most overweight people are also chronically inflamed—the crucial factor that makes obesity trigger chronic diseases. This manifests in the mouth in the form of inflamed gums, but is also a risk factor for almost all other chronic diseases.

In addition, those who are obese make less adiponectin and leptin. A lack of these substances leads to a higher level of insulin, which in turn leads to insulin resistance in the long term and consequently, diabetes mellitus (type 2 diabetes), which in turn is related to periodontitis. Low leptin levels have another harmful effect. Leptin has an impact on bone remodeling and aids in bone growth via the hypothalamus while simultaneously stimulating osteoblasts, the cells that aid in bone formation. For strong teeth and bones, the body therefore needs sufficient levels of leptin to help keep fat cell counts low. This also means the anti-inflammatory effects of leptin are washed down the drain. So obesity promotes the inflammatory tendencies of the body, which not only is noticeable in the mouth, but can harm the entire organism. A body with a high fat content is therefore always an inflamed body. When we get rid of fat, we also get rid of the stress and strain on the body caused by chronic inflammation. Even an insulin resistance can be completely reversed by losing weight.

## Diabetes Mellitus

If there were a prize for the chronic disease that develops the quickest, diabetes mellitus would be number one on the podium. Around seven million people suffer from this metabolic disease in Germany alone. People often believe that diabetes is the result of having too much sugar in the body. It would be more correct to say that it's the result of not being able to get rid of the sugar in the body. The sugar molecules need to end up in our (muscle) cells to give us energy. For this to happen, cells need to allow this process to occur, and the hormone insulin needs to help them by opening up the cells and pushing the molecules in.

In certain people the pancreas stops insulin production at a young age, and they need to inject insulin to be able to ingest sugar. This form of diabetes is referred to as type 1 and is usually genetically determined or epigenetic—caused by an unfavorable adaptation to the conditions in our environment. The other type of diabetes is type 2. Until recently this was also considered age-related diabetes, because it mainly occurred in older people and was thought to be caused by deterioration. In fact, this form of diabetes affects the receptivity of the cells to insulin while simultaneously decreasing the production of insulin. Today the term *age-related diabetes* has become practically obsolete, because increasingly young patients are being diagnosed with the disease. There is little doubt that diabetes is primarily a diet and lifestyle disease. The cells and pancreases of increasing numbers of people are simply giving up in light of the ever-increasing torrent of simple carbohydrates and the constant sugar spikes they cause.

Next up on the winner's podium for nasty, fast-acting diseases would be periodontitis. These two diseases develop at roughly the same pace—which is no coincidence. Diabetes and periodontitis are best buddies and have quite a significant mutual impact. They happily play ping-pong in the patient's body, making them increasingly sick. There is strong evidence that centers of inflammation in the mouth increase the insulin resistance of cells and thus contribute to the decrease in blood sugar levels.[2] High blood sugar levels stimulate the body to release more insulin, and high insulin levels in turn favor inflammation, which, as we have seen, aggravates periodontitis. Anyone looking for a textbook example of a vicious circle will quickly find it in the interplay between periodontitis and diabetes.

But this negative spiral can quickly be reversed and made into a positive one. When diabetes patients get rid of inflammation centers in the mouth, their sugar levels also improve. The better adjusted a diabetic's sugar levels are, the better their overall health will be. The more constant the blood sugar levels of a diabetic are, the lower their risk of getting one of the more serious complications of diabetes. It's always worthwhile for diabetics to fine-tune their diets and keep their blood sugar levels constant. Diabetes has long been considered incurable. But today we know that we can make considerable improvements with the right diet, often to such an extent that those with diabetes no longer need insulin injections. Studies suggest that diabetes can be treated just as well with diet and weight loss as with medication.

A diet that keeps insulin levels low isn't only recommended for diabetics—it can be beneficial for anyone. Above all, it helps to prevent diabetes, because if we can be certain of one thing, it's that diabetes doesn't simply fall from the sky. It's a silent killer. Many people live for a long time in what is known as a prediabetic metabolic state before they are given an official diagnosis. Even at this stage glucose tolerance is significantly disrupted, which creates favorable conditions for heart attacks, stroke, blindness, kidney failure, and nerve damage. According to estimates by the National Institute of Diabetes and Digestive and Kidney Diseases in the United States, almost fifty-seven million adults in Europe currently have prediabetes, which is also known as insulin resistance.

## Allergies

Our immune system has two different sides: One side eyes anything foreign suspiciously whenever it feels threatened. But it also has a tolerant side that's at least as important. Perhaps the best way to imagine the immune system is as a stern bouncer.

When dangerous-looking characters turn up, it gives off unmistakable signs to let these types know they should clear off. Meanwhile, all other guests are waved through. The success of the venue always depends on the security's ability to effectively assess each guest. The venue relies on visitors, but it's important that trouble stays outside. Our immune system works best when it is able to recognize and fight harmful influences and leave harmless visitors in peace. But it's precisely this last characteristic that the immune system is increasingly starting to lose.

To understand why this is the case, we have to take a closer look at the working conditions of our immunological bouncer. The immune system, which is primarily responsible for getting rid of viruses, fungi, bacteria, and other microorganisms, now has to deal with so many foreign substances and stimuli that it is starting to lose its overview of the situation. Humans and their immune systems have always had to adapt to changing environmental conditions over the course of their evolution. Today, however, these changes are taking place at such a fast pace that the organism can barely keep up. Our personal bouncer is therefore forced to relinquish its more tolerant side. The situation in front of the door has become so confusing that the bouncer becomes overcautious and scares away not only attackers, but also those standing in front of the door with a pressed shirt and a bouquet of flowers in hand.

We can tell this is happening when, for example, after eating a certain type of food, we suddenly feel a little bit sick or bloated, or notice an itchy rash. But unfortunately the link isn't always immediately obvious, so people search for a long time in vain for the cause of their symptoms.

Every living being on earth has an immune system, but we humans also have a bonus function: Not only do we have a general immune system, we also have a specific one. The specific immune system is able to perform the one trick all good bouncers need to have up their sleeve: If someone has caused trouble before, remember their face forever. This is why, when someone gets a sneezing attack just once under a hazel tree, they continue to have the same attacks like clockwork at the same time each year. At the first sign of pollen, the memory cells have spotted it on their radar and the bouncer is already standing outside with his arms folded. Normally our organism should be able to cope well with the absorption and inhalation of all sorts

## Material Allergies

The body reacts to many foreign substances in the mouth with an allergy. Common triggers include eugenol, Peru balsam, and rosin. Even printing materials can be allergenic or put the body in a situation that makes it more sensitive to certain substances. Chronic inflammation also contributes to making the organism more prone to allergies and autoimmune diseases. In the midst of chronic inflammatory processes, the immune system's tolerance function gradually gets lost. Humans can also be allergic to bacterial toxins, especially toxins such as thioethers and mercaptans, which are typically found in teeth that have undergone root canal treatment. Symptoms rarely appear locally, but when they do, they might manifest in the form of reddened or bleeding gums. Much more often, sufferers experience systemic symptoms such as fatigue, exhaustion, or increased susceptibility to infections.

of natural substances. But if house dust, grass, or food causes us to constantly look like we've just peeled an onion, that's a clear sign that our doorman has had enough and become rather intolerant. An allergy is therefore simply an overreaction of the immune system when everything becomes too much for it. But an allergy doesn't necessarily mean a rash or streaming eyes. Symptoms can manifest in all manner of ways, for example through depression, a lack of motivation, or constantly getting infections. Only around 30 percent of people notice an intolerance to the grain component gluten in the gastrointestinal tract. The remaining 70 percent experience symptoms of a different nature—usually neurological.

The teeth and mouth are very often the decisive area that determines whether the immune system becomes hypersensitive or not.

When metals, chronic inflammation, or toxins affect our immune and nervous systems twenty-four hours a day without interruption, the body creates an environment that greatly increases the body's intolerance. There is simply too much going on.

Most dental materials were developed at a time when the focus was only on functionality. Today we know that many materials have a strong potential to make the organism sick. Nowadays tools don't only have to work well; they must also take the patient's organism into account. Fortunately, there are many materials available today that do this, so there is no need to resort to these problematic materials (see "The Right Treatment for Dead and Root-Treated Teeth" on page 121).

Time and again in my practice, I watch as my patients' immune systems become more tolerant once triggers are removed. Once metals are removed from the mouth, for example, relieving the burden on the system, patients are able to tolerate things that have been problematic for them in the past.

## Autoimmune Diseases

Sometimes things get to be too much for the immune system, and it turns against not only those standing in front of the door, but the domestic staff as well. The immune system can usually distinguish which cells are foreign and which belong to our bodies. This is because every single cell in the human body carries a certain mark that shows the immune system it has the right to be there. But when the immune system is in crisis mode, it sometimes loses the ability to recognize this mark and starts to attack the body's own cells. The immune system's defense cells then proceed to attack, for example, skin, bone, organs, or nerve cells. Healthy tissues become damaged, and the affected areas remain permanently inflamed. At this point, the problem is no longer referred to as an allergy, but as an autoimmune disease.

The system that should be protecting us actually turns against us. In this kind of situation, many chronic diseases such as multiple sclerosis, rheumatoid arthritis, type 1 diabetes, and chronic inflammatory bowel diseases like Crohn's disease or ulcerative colitis begin to take their course. Over four million people suffer from autoimmune diseases in Germany alone. The risk factors for the mouth and allergies are the same. But autoimmune diseases also frequently start in the gut. There is some discussion about a possible connection between autoimmune diseases and toxins that accumulate or are stored in the body's own cells, and are therefore flagged by the immune system as foreign (the carrier effect).

## A Disrupted Intestinal Barrier: Leaky Gut Syndrome

If you wanted to give someone a truly unsolvable task, you might ask them to do the following: Create a barrier that is both permeable and tightly sealed at the same time. It's quite a challenge. Yet our gut manages to create such a barrier with ease. After all, it constantly has to find everything that is valuable and useful and let it pass through its walls, while rejecting all it finds harmful or useless.

The secret mechanisms behind this magic barrier are known as tight junctions. These are special cell-to-cell connections that make

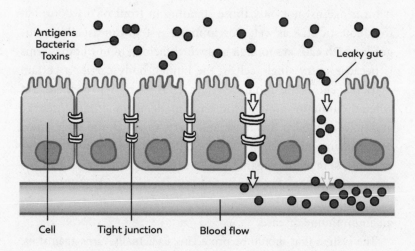

**Figure 3.2.** Tight junctions.

up the intestinal wall. Within this area, plasma proteins stay very close together. The connection between neighboring cells works like a ziplock. This makes the intestinal wall so dense that it can protect the inside of our bodies from external influences, while remaining permeable to the nutrients that we need to live.

Certain factors, however, cause these connections to loosen and rupture. One of these factors is gluten, a component of many cereal products. The syndrome can also be brought on by stress that irritates the intestine and blocks the immune system, metals in the mouth, or a disruption to the oral flora that makes us permanently swallow toxins or the wrong groups of bacteria. If the spaces between the cells grow larger, this increases the permeability of the intestinal wall. As a result, not only can important nutrients slip through, but so can antigens, bacteria, toxins, or undigested food residues. This is a red alert for the intestine and the organism as a whole. The best-case scenario is that the immune system—which largely resides in our intestines—will react with local inflammation. But this can increase the permeability of the tight junction even further, allowing even more foreign substances to enter and continue to fuel the inflammation, once again creating a vicious circle.

However, leaky gut syndrome can also mark the beginning of an autoimmune process in which the immune system is no longer able to clearly differentiate between its own and foreign body cells and therefore begins to damage its own cells. In the end so many substances enter the body unchecked that it's impossible to know where to go first to eliminate them. This kind of environment can cause all kinds of problems. These include hay fever and allergies, but also autoimmune diseases such as Hashimoto's thyroiditis, multiple sclerosis, and rheumatoid arthritis.

Our gut needs to be well at all times and it's at its best when we eat the right things. If we eat the right diet, we let our gut know that it can leave us in peace. A stomach that only has to digest good, wholesome food does so without a fuss. Whenever we experience flatulence, feel constantly bloated, or notice anything happening in our stomachs, it's an indication that the bowel is having issues. I explain what sort of nutrition is good for the body (and soul) in chapter 4.

## From Sparks to Wildfire

If we continue to eat things that cause inflammation every day or have permanent inflammation triggers in our mouths, it's a bit like pouring gasoline onto the same spot every day—and the spot in question isn't as small as you might think. If you were to roll out the entire length of your gut, it would take up an area as large as two tennis courts.

## Depression

Depression can be a terrible ordeal. Because the symptoms are primarily psychological, doctors tend to try to understand and treat it from a psychological perspective. It's widely considered that harmful or traumatic events in a person's past can lead to the development of depression. Grief, losing important people in one's life, abuse, or mistreatment can take their toll on a person's psyche. Nevertheless, recent research has also begun to explore the physical causes of depression. The focus of this research—much like the focus of this book—has been on inflammatory markers such as interleukin and tumor necrosis factors, which are released when the body is fighting inflammation. Scientists have noticed that in almost all chronic diseases involving inflammation, such as diabetes (type 2), rheumatism, multiple sclerosis, and inflammatory bowel disease, a large number of patients also suffer from depression.[3] One might argue that those who are suffering from a serious illness are more likely to be stressed. But today we know that people are not just psychologically responsive to their conditions; a large part of depression is due to biological factors.

Anyone who has had a flu infection will have had a tiny sample of this mechanism in action. Nobody can jump around the room or go partying after the flu. This is because when the immune system is stretched, it wants us to shut down so that it can do its work better in peace. This is why "sickness behavior" is triggered when we are unwell. This syndrome makes us feel unwell and unmotivated; it makes us lose our appetite, and we become completely disinterested in the world for a while. From a biological point of view, it makes sense in this kind of situation to feel this way for a short period of time. But problems arise when the cause persists and this feeling of depression becomes a permanent state. The cause can be any form of chronic inflammation in the body, including in the mouth—say, an inflamed tooth root, NICOs, or diseased gums.

A recent study found a clear link between inflamed root tips (and the toxins they release) and major depression. According to the study, this type of inflammation can cause "depression and a diminished quality of life." Later on, the study states that such teeth are "closely related to the aetiology and course of depression and significantly affect a person's quality of life."[4] The emergence and development of depression can also begin in the mouth.

Another factor our system uses to respond to inflammation and metal toxins is stress. Stress can knock us for six and give us long-term anxiety because it releases a constant flow of cortisol. Certain sections of our brains are particularly sensitive to cortisol. It is well known that certain cells of the hippocampus die under the influence of cortisol. The hippocampus is the part of the brain that has a calming effect on us and ensures that grief and anxiety do not get out of hand. But its soothing voice gets drowned out in the flood of cortisol. Psychologically, this manifests as fears, worries, mental loops, and negative thoughts. This can also trigger symptoms that fit the diagnosis criteria for anxiety. The end result is that depression often increases the original symptoms. A person experiencing a depressive episode has less energy and motivation to look after themselves and take care to get the right nutrition and sufficient exercise. They often neglect a healthy lifestyle and sometimes even oral hygiene. In addition, stress and antibiotic treatments also decrease salivation, which causes more problems in the mouth.

## Fertility and Childbearing

More and more couples are finding themselves unable to have children for long periods of time—sometimes their whole lives. A confusingly wide range of specialized facilities and new fertility treatments have cropped up in answer to this problem. Yet too often, the influence that problems in the mouth can have on fertility and childbirth is overlooked. Inflammation in the mouth is associated with the metabolic and hormonal disease PCOS, as well as endometriosis, bacterial vaginosis, gestational diabetes, preeclampsia, preterm birth, and low birth weight.[5]

The risk of having an underweight, premature baby was increased sevenfold in studies of pregnant women with severe periodontitis. Australian doctors specializing in reproductive health found in an observational study with 3,737 participants that women with periodontitis needed seven instead of the usual five months to get pregnant. Links have also been found between male infertility and oral health.

Stress also plays a huge role. Many couples who have been trying for a long time often hear: "Just relax, it will work out in the end." There is some truth to this, because when the body's nervous and hormonal systems are at war or MIA, the body doesn't usually like to reproduce. Sometimes, though, doing more yoga or switching off after work simply isn't enough. It's also important to take into account the stress that may arise from the inside due to chronic inflammation in the mouth that could go unnoticed. Once inflammation and any metals are removed, the organism, including the hormone system, is finally able to rest. In particular, women who are affected by the hormone imbalance PCOS can benefit from a good diet that stabilizes blood sugar levels and therefore lowers insulin secretion.

## Alzheimer's and Dementia

Scientists still don't have a clear answer as to what exactly causes Alzheimer's and other forms of dementia. What is clear is that these diseases are always accompanied by inflammatory processes in the brain. In many recent studies in which scientists looked closely at the brains of Alzheimer's patients, they kept coming across bacteria that would usually be found elsewhere—in an inflamed mouth—alongside the typical protein deposits. The authors of the study point out that

## Denture Danger

One of the factors that can increase the risk of Alzheimer's may be hiding under some patients' removable dentures. Dentures often harbor large quantities of oral candida, a sort of fungus, as well as the bacteria responsible for denture-related stomatitis and inflammation of the oral mucosa. Another study has linked denture-related stomatitis and systemic fungal infections with Alzheimer's.[6]

the inflammatory changes in the brains of those affected may also be associated with inflammation in the mouth.[7]

Researchers believe that bacteria travel from the mouth to other parts of the body as a result of normal processes such as chewing or brushing teeth. Usually they are quickly stopped on the way to the rest of the organism by a healthy immune system. If they find their way to the brain, they are usually stopped by a particularly stringent border control: the blood-brain barrier. However, it appears that an excess of microorganisms affects the blood-brain barrier, especially in the elderly, making it easy for microbes to invade and destroy nerve tissue. Metals also play a role in neurodegenerative (brain damaging) diseases. Mercury in particular accumulates in the nerve tissue and is known to destroy certain nerve cell structures.

## Cancer

Most people know that the immune system protects us from foreign bodies and influences. But fewer people know about how it maintains the order in our bodies by keeping in check any degenerate cells that could potentially grow into a tumor. Macrophages, our diligent Pac-Man-like cells, play a particularly big role in this process. When they encounter cells that are out of line, they solve the problem in their usual way: They eliminate the intruders by eating them, killing them with special molecules or calling in other immune cells to organize a coordinated attack against the tumor. They then present parts of the degenerate cells to the rest of the system, thereby activating the acquired immune response against the tumor.

Studies are currently exploring the connection between chronic inflammation and the development of cancer, because scientists have found that the presence of chronic inflammation impairs the mechanism described above. It has also been proven that an inflamed organism provides the best conditions for tumors to thrive in.[8]

There is evidence that tumors develop strategies to sustain the body's ongoing state of battle by releasing inflammatory factors themselves. By doing so, not only do they provide better conditions for themselves to thrive in, they also manipulate the immune system's defense cells—the cells that should normally be responsible for fighting them. If defense cells are permanently programmed to cause inflammation, they sometimes even provide the tumor with the necessary fuel for its growth. This whole process can go so far that the function of the defense cells is completely reversed because they prevent the immune cells from taking targeted action to fight the tumor.

This is partly due to the fact that macrophages in our body are mainly there as progenitor cells. If they were part of a police operation, we might imagine them as students of the police force. But while real police students have to spend a long time in school to prepare for all the different types of criminals they are likely to encounter, progenitor cells learn on the job. They only specialize in one type of crime, and that's the crime that they come into contact with at any given time. The role of a macrophage also depends on which signals it receives from the cells it encounters and other immune cells.

Some tumor cells master the deceptive little trick of sending signals to these police students to tell them that they need help rather than to be destroyed. Macrophages then actually begin helping these cells, attracting more immune cells and even keeping their surrounding environment inflamed. Research is currently under way to reveal more of these cells' tricks. One thing we are sure of is that there is a possibility we can prevent or weaken cancer by curing chronic inflammation or leading lifestyles that do not cause chronic inflammation in the first place.

One of the cells that is suspected of being involved in the development of cancer is the immune messenger RANTES, also known as CCL5.

## The Key to a Healthy Life

It is quite clear what role the mouth plays in the development of many serious diseases. But it is important that we don't overlook the message behind this fact: If disease in the mouth can create the right conditions for these problems, a healthy mouth can reduce problems or ensure they never arise in the first place. When it comes to disease, especially chronic disease, we too often overlook the fact that diseases are not an inevitable fate; there are also measures we can take to help cure them. Sometimes, doctors themselves are the ones who overlook this fact.

The dilemma is that a disease often begins with a diagnosis. A diagnosis gives a patient an explanation for their problems—but this always comes with a big extra helping of fear: the fear that we will never be well or quite the same again. In certain cases people begin to identify with or define themselves by their diagnosis. This is partly because our health care system is focused on diseases. It relieves symptoms but rarely shows us how the causes of a disease can be treated. Often the diagnosis is the only information a patient receives, along with—at best—the list of medicines they now have to take.

Many people therefore become trapped in their diseases. This goes on for so long that they are hardly able to believe they can take matters into their own hands. There are usually things patients can do for themselves. Our bodies have an enormous amount of regenerative power. When we get to the bottom of what is causing a disease and start treating our bodies properly, many things can start to change. I am meeting more and more patients who believe in this—people who belong to a new health consciousness and who are setting out to find solutions to their problems. I see the health of my patients improving every day in my practice when the cause of their problems is properly treated. Few chronic diseases are the result of a simple stroke of fate that we must simply succumb to and accept. There are solutions for many problems, and often they begin in a place we rarely pay attention to: our mouths.

# Get Healthy and Stay Healthy with Biological Dentistry

E veryone is capable of making changes to make great improvements to their health. We can start by eating differently, reducing the amount of stress we have in our daily lives, and focusing on the things that are good for us. But when our organisms are under significant strain that is firmly established in the mouth and is taking effect 24/7, they need extra help. Biological dentistry may just be the piece of the puzzle we need for a healthier life. Our mouths are the gateway to the rest of the body. Whatever happens in the mouth, gets transported from the mouth, or has an impact on the mouth also has an impact on the rest of the body.

Biological dentistry is well aware of this. It isn't about repairing one tooth after the next, but about making the body as healthy as possible by freeing it from anything that is likely to disturb it, poison it, or make it ill. This realization can be the salvation of chronically ill people. For others, it can simply be a step toward better efficiency. As soon as chronic inflammation is removed from the body, the overactive immune system is relieved, or metals are taken away, the body often feels as though it's finally able to breathe again. Often it then switches to the parasympathetic mode, the only program in which the immune system is able to function properly and regeneration can take place. Many patients experience this state for the first time in years following treatment and feel a significant change. But first things first . . .

## Removal of Metals

Because of the enormous immunological and toxicological strain they place the organism under, metals no longer have a place in the mouth. All metals should be removed from the mouth as part of thorough biological dentistry treatment. But this procedure should only take place under careful protective measures. There is one metal in particular that requires very strict protective measures: amalgam.

### Removal of Amalgam

Unfortunately, it is precisely when patients seek to have their amalgam fillings removed that most mistakes happen. Many dentists are still too careless when dealing with amalgam. Those who are not aware of the problems related to amalgam (see "Metals in the Mouth? Never the Right Solution" on page 69) may not see the need to take any special protective measures when removing it. As a result, some dentists put in danger not only their patients, but also themselves. In my first few years working as a dentist, I protected my patients, but out of ignorance I didn't think to protect myself.

Now when I remove amalgam in my practice, the room looks a little bit like a space center. Because large quantities of highly toxic, inorganic mercury vapor are released during the drilling process to remove amalgam fillings, this procedure can only take place under maximum protective conditions.

Some of the protective measures I use in my practice include:

- Rubber dam: This protective rubber cloth is inserted over the teeth and covers right up to the back of the mouth. This protects the mouth from chips and fragments.
- Cleanup suction tube: This provides extra protection from mercury vapors.
- Careful drilling: Amalgam must be removed with the dental handpiece (also known as a dental drill) set at a low speed to avoid toxic mercury vapor from escaping. Ideally, the filling should be drilled in such a way that the majority can be taken out in one go, which prevents vapor being released in the first place.

## To Remove or Not to Remove?

Practically any dentist can remove amalgam, but few carry out the procedure using adequate protective measures. If a dentist does not take the measures outlined in this chapter, they should not be carrying out the procedure. This is because most problems arise as a result of improper removal of amalgam. But this is no reason for keeping fillings containing mercury where they are. It is always better to remove the constant toxic burden amalgam puts the body under—and it should always be removed by someone using the appropriate protective measures.

- Fresh air supply via a nasal probe.
- Air purifier: A special air purifier such as the IQAir can remove up to 99 percent of mercury vapor in the air. This is good for both the patient and doctor.
- A dentist should always wear an additional FFP3 protective mask, which filters 99 percent of invisible mercury vapor.
- The insertion of a chlorella algae insert once the amalgam has been removed absorbs any leftover mercury.

## The Right Treatment for Dead and Root-Treated Teeth

Two things biological dentists do not like to see are dead teeth and teeth that have undergone root canal treatment. This is not just a whim of biological dentists; outside of dentistry, no other medical discipline tolerates dead body parts being left in the body. They are removed as quickly as possible because of the inflammation they can cause and toxic risks they pose. Root canal treatment can initially provide relief and certainly contributes to the disinfection process in the short term. But sooner or later, a dead or root-canal-treated tooth will be repopulated with bacteria and, as a result, will always lead to chronic problems in the body. From a biological dentistry perspective, a root canal treatment should only ever be used as acute pain treatment. But if you've had root canal treatment, this isn't to say you need to panic. There's no rush to remove every root-treated tooth immediately. That said, I recommend that anyone who has undergone treatment be critically questioned and examined for signs of inflammation or cysts at the root tips. A healthy body can usually tolerate chronic inflammation for a while until another solution is found. When looking for a solution to this issue, it is always important to take into account the patient's overall health and what their goals are. Do they need to be at the top of their game and stay completely healthy? Are they experiencing any discomfort or is the tooth bothering them because it is discolored and aesthetically unpleasant? For chronically ill people and high-performance athletes, I recommend finding a suitable doctor who can remove the diseased tooth, thoroughly clean and disinfect the surrounding structures, and as a bonus replace the tooth with a ceramic implant.

## Ceramic Implants: The Metal-Free Solution

Despite low success rates, root canal treatments have prevailed for so long because there has been no good alternative available. The other option was pulling the tooth out and inserting a dental bridge into the gap, which can later be filled with a titanium implant. As long as there is a hint of a chance of saving a tooth, most dentists will take it and do everything they can to make sure the tooth survives. This is because dentists are traditionally trained to preserve teeth—and who wouldn't be happy to hear: "We can save the tooth!" The fact that saving a tooth can sometimes be at the expense of the patient's overall health, however, is often overlooked. Biological medicine sees things the other way around. We don't talk of teeth being sacrificed. Dentistry, technology, and implantology have made enormous progress in recent years. Diseased teeth can cause serious chronic diseases, but removing them has historically come at a high cost: Loss of bone and gums, unpleasant aesthetics, comfort, time, money, and self-confidence were all at stake. Today things are different because new, highly biocompatible materials are available. In biological dentistry, ceramic implants are the material of choice when it comes to filling a gap. If you're wondering, "But does ceramic stay put?"—don't worry. The material is a world apart from Grandma's tea set. Today we use high-performance ceramic made from zirconium (di)oxide, which surpasses metals in terms of stability and, above all, biocompatibility.

One of the pioneers in the field of metal-free dentistry is my friend and colleague Dr. Ulrich Volz. He decided very early on to do away with metal completely when treating his patients. In 2001 he developed a metal-free ceramic implant. Now ceramics are on the rise more than any other material in dentistry, yet only around 1 percent of implantologists use it. Zirconium oxide implants do not conduct heat, which means the surgeon has to focus more on the condition of the bones. Additionally, they can only heal in a healthy body with healthy bones, which means the dentist carrying out the treatment needs to be very familiar with the correct healing process. Aside from these two constraints, there are many advantages to ceramic implants. Unlike gray titanium, they are free from metal and completely white. The dreaded gray edges that always show up sooner

## Bridging the Gap . . . Unsuccessfully

Often a tooth gap is filled with what is known as a dental bridge as a cheaper alternative to an implant. But bridges come at a high biological price. Because the tooth replacement is inserted into the gap between neighboring teeth, the teeth on either side have to be contoured. The patient therefore loses a significant amount of healthy tooth. Contouring teeth also puts them at risk of damage; the teeth can even die during the procedure, causing a potential problem in itself.

or later on a conventional crown or implant become a thing of the past with ceramic. But the most crucial factor for biological dentists is that they are completely neutral (as long as they aren't dyed): They do not release electrons and therefore don't cause interference in the body. Ceramic is also very friendly to the body's tissues. Unlike metal materials, the gums are able to grow properly around ceramic, which heals well in the bone and accumulates less plaque. This in turn helps to counteract inflammation.

## A Guide to Treating NICOs

Wherever wisdom teeth have been removed—especially if the extraction took place during puberty—it is likely that chronically inflamed extraction wounds have developed, which dentists like to call NICOs (see "NICOs: Wisdom Tooth Extraction and Its Consequences" on page 61). Anyone who is curious about NICOs can ask their dentist for a panoramic image (an X-ray), followed by a DVT 3-D X-ray. However, it's important to go to a dentist who is familiar with NICOs and able to recognize their pathological structures. Dentists who are not trained to spot NICOs will not be able to find them on an X-ray. On the positive side, those who are able to identify NICOs are also able to treat them.

NICOs can be removed using a minimally invasive surgical technique. The wound is cleaned out and disinfected with ozone using hand tools and a technique known as Piezosurgery, a procedure carried out with the help of ultrasound. In my practice the wound area is then filled with APRF membranes. This is a biological material made from the patient's own blood, which makes it highly natural and biocompatible. The procedure therefore draws upon a mechanism that the body would usually use to heal itself. When the human body is injured, it generates proteins to accelerate the wound healing process. These can then be used for the production of natural tissues. A small amount of blood is taken from the patient and centrifuged then used to make a suspension fluid with a high concentration of platelets. These platelets contain information required for tissue regeneration. When these are placed in the wounded area of the

## Immediate Implants

When a tooth needs to be removed, a dentist usually has to wait a while for the wound to heal before filling the gap with an implant. But it turns out that doing the opposite is actually much more effective. Once the tooth is out, it's best to insert the implant immediately, because this ensures that the bone and soft tissues are supported right away. An implant acts like a kind of plug that supports the tooth socket and bone. In addition, the body's regeneration capacity is at its highest when the tooth is removed, since the body is trying to heal the wound anyway. At this time, there are more growth factors being released and protein synthesis is running at full speed. The body also has to rebuild fewer bones this way, because the implant takes up a certain amount of space itself. If there is an extended period of time between the tooth extraction and implant insertion, it's often the case that valuable bone substance is lost and has to be rebuilt.

treated NICO, they serve as a matrix for bone regeneration and also stimulate tissue regeneration.

### The Importance of Preparation Before Surgery

The general practice in dentistry is to operate on people more or less as they come in off the street. The only preparation for surgery or any other invasive procedure is premedication or information about the treatment. The procedure therefore comes as a shock to the body. Most postoperative traumas such as swelling, pain, and inflammation are not just side effects of the operation; they are above all evidence that the body is not able to compensate for the procedure.

Most people living in the Western world are in immunological hibernation. Many of us are poorly nourished because our eating habits and the way in which our food is prepared are no longer adequate, and in winter we don't get enough sun to make vitamin D. Any surgical procedure puts the body under tremendous stress and requires a great deal of healing. This is particularly true for dental and jaw surgeries, which require a special pre-op procedure. To make sure my patients are able to compensate for the stress caused by surgery and optimize the regeneration process to avoid failure or recurrence, they are instructed to prepare for the procedure according to a specific protocol.

Anything that could prevent bone regeneration after a tooth extraction—or the healing of the interference field or implant—is prohibited. This means, in particular, that patients should pay attention to nutrition and avoid high quantities of sugar, wheat, or dairy products, as well as ensuring they are not deficient in any vitamins or nutrients. Before the surgery phase, the patient's diet should be as hypoallergenic and anti-inflammatory as possible, while remaining high in nutrients. When our bodies are deficient in vitamin $D_3$, minerals (zinc and magnesium), trace minerals, omega-3 fatty acids, and other micronutrients, the body is overwhelmed by the combination of the deficiency and the healing process.

This means it's unable to build new tissue because it simply lacks the nutrients it needs to do so. This is why we encourage every patient to ensure they get the right (micro)nutrients and nutrition. This isn't important only for people undergoing a surgical procedure—it should be practiced by everyone at all times. The best thing a person can do for their teeth and overall health is to eat well. Because nutrition is so immensely important but at the same time, extremely complicated, I have developed my own concepts to make it easy for people to eat well and stay healthily.

## The Healing Power of Nutrition

*The food you eat can either be the safest and most*
*powerful form of medicine or the slowest form of poison.*

—Ann Wigmore, nutrition expert

Hardly any other factor affects our health as much as the food we consume. Yet the subject receives hardly any attention in the field of medicine. As Ann Wigmore puts it, the food we eat can either cure or poison us. It's astounding how little doctors in training learn about nutrition at school. During their studies, dentists, who get to see firsthand the consequences of poor nutrition, are not even prepared to advise patients what sort of diet would be most beneficial for them. "Avoid snacking between meals" more or less sums up the information we are given, which usually goes in one ear and out the other. Treatment concepts that don't take nutrition into account are a bit like an attempt to build a house without laying down the foundations first. But in the past we were much more clued up on nutrition. More than two thousand years ago, Hippocrates's motto was as follows: "Let food be thy medicine and medicine be thy food." Unfortunately, it would appear that this motto has now been forgotten. If we think about it, it seems as though the opposite is in fact true: The average Western diet makes us sick rather than healthy.

Nutrition is a key factor in biological dentistry. The nutritional model I have designed takes foods in their purest form as the basis for all biochemical processes in the body. It's a kind of medicine for healing purposes and is designed to make people healthy and strong in the long term. I believe that nutrition should be the basis for all forms of therapy. This doesn't mean following a short-term diet, calorie counting, or giving up foods. It's about starting a new lifestyle and making long-term changes, which are critical factors in helping people get well on all levels—physically, mentally, and emotionally.

The standard Western diet consists mainly of wheat, dairy products, sugar, and processed foods, of which there is an infinite selection in supermarkets. Above all, there is a wide range of refined and processed foods containing a high quantity of simple sugars, along with the types of fats that are bad for us, flavor enhancers, and sometimes chemical sweeteners. Our body processes these kinds of artificial combinations of foods differently from natural foods. There is no such thing as a pizza tree in nature. The combination of fats and starchy carbohydrates is unnatural. Industrially produced food manipulates our metabolism and above all, our innate instincts and feeling of satiety. If we generally eat high-quality, natural products, on the other hand, hunger and satiety can regulate themselves. It's not very often that someone has a craving for eggs and eats twelve at a time. But it's not uncommon for people to eat two pizzas, followed by three scoops of ice cream and a Coke. Eighty percent of the things you can buy at the supermarket are not healthy. Gluten, dairy products, trans fats, additives, and flavor enhancers can lead to dietary intolerances and are sometimes actually poisonous to our bodies, which is why they are known as nutritional toxins. These foods trigger inflammation in the body, as well as stress in the nervous system, making us sick and overweight in the long term.

Medicine, as I understand it, needs to provide people everything they need to care for themselves and optimize their health. This is why I've broken down the complex topic of nutrition to its absolute basics, so that anyone can easily create their own nutrition plan. My nutritional model dispels myths and false information about nutrition. It can help anyone incorporate long-term diet and lifestyle changes into their daily routines, providing them with the right nutrients and optimal health, fitness, and balance. And all this without pesky calorie counting and the other stresses that come with being on a diet.

Excess body fat goes away by itself over time as the metabolism kicks in again. Bodily functions such as digestion, detoxification, and excretion run at full speed. Nutrition deficiencies are corrected, cells regenerate, and bones, muscles, skin, hair, and nails all get stronger. Within just one year the entire body rebuilds itself completely, and this new lifestyle makes it healthier, fitter, and even slimmer and more attractive. A lifestyle based on healthy, nutritious food can be seen as a comprehensive provision for the future. Generally people don't feel as though they are giving anything up, but instead feel the relief of unburdening themselves of unhealthy things. At the beginning this requires a little bit of discipline, but usually after just a few days we start to feel a positive change and feel bad if we eat the foods that our diets previously consisted of.

The following section provides some basic information to help simplify the topic of nutrition.

## Why Calorie Counting Is Not Effective

Calories are physical units, also known as calorific values. The term indicates the specific energy in foods that is released as a result of the body's metabolism process. However, biochemistry is not taken into account as part of this energy calculation. Here's a simple example: A bottle of Coca-Cola contains as many calories as a handful of almonds. The calories in Coke come exclusively from sugar, while the calories in the portion of almonds are made up of healthy fats, long-chain carbohydrates, and a small amount of protein and fiber. While blood sugar levels rise to a maximum within minutes due to the consumption of Coke and a lot of insulin is released, the nutrients in the portion of almonds are released slowly and steadily over a long period of time. Blood sugar levels remain almost constant throughout this process. The number of calories is the same but the effects of the food on the metabolism and therefore on feelings of hunger and fitness levels differ considerably.

### Protein

The word *protein* comes from the Greek word *proteus*, meaning "first" and "most important." Proteins play a crucial role in the human body and are involved in numerous functions. They are the most important raw material for building and repairing cells, such as those that make up our hair, skin, muscles, and nerves. But they are also involved in the body's detoxification and excretion processes. Every enzyme is made up of the amino acids contained in protein, which means protein is of paramount importance for the metabolism. Those eating a conventional diet are usually deficient in protein, and therefore in amino acids. But in times of increased requirements in particular, such as after surgery or during a detoxification phase, it is important to make sure we get a particularly high amount of protein.

## Good Sources of Protein

**Plant-Based Protein**

CHLORELLA: This freshwater algae is a superfood containing sixty grams of protein per hundred-gram portion, with a complete amino acid profile.

GRAINS: Quinoa, sometimes referred to as the power corn of the Incas, contains a complete amino acid profile, making it equivalent in nutritional value to animal products.

NUTS: All unsalted nuts such as almonds, Brazil nuts, walnuts, cashews, hazelnuts, macadamia nuts, pecans, pistachios, and pine nuts. *Note:* Peanuts are not classed as nuts, but as legumes, and commonly cause allergies.

SEEDS: Pumpkin, sesame, hemp, and sunflower seeds.

SOY: Is generally not recommended. Exceptions include fermented products such as miso, natto, and tempeh. Look for the "non-GMO" label for products that are not genetically modified.

LEGUMES: Peas, beans, and lentils. These are relatively rich in amino acids but do not have a complete profile. Ideal for vegans. *Note:* Allergies to legumes are common because not everyone is able to digest them properly.

**Animal Proteins**

BEEF: Generally speaking, red meat has a bad reputation. The problem here is the way in which the cow is raised. Grass-fed pasture cattle is one of the best sources of anti-inflammatory omega-3 fatty acids and high-quality protein, putting it among the superfoods. Factory farming, however, feeds cattle on wheat, corn, and concentrated feed, creating the beautiful marbling effect that is much desired among consumers but is unfortunately transforming beef into a highly inflammatory product. Lean variants (a fat content below 18 percent) are better for our health.

**EGGS:** Eggs are the most bioavailable source of protein. Egg yolks contain important phospholipids, which are essential for the development of nerve sheaths. Egg yolks are best consumed runny, for example soft-boiled. Only organic eggs should be purchased.

**FISH:** Fish has also gained something of a bad reputation, and there are many people who just don't like it. But high-quality fish contains plenty of healthy protein and numerous omega-3 fatty acids. The larger the fish variety (tuna, swordfish), the more toxins accumulate in the fatty tissues (especially heavy metals). The varieties I mostly recommend are salmon (Alaskan wild salmon), cod, gilthead sea bream, sea bass, and small fish such as sardines and mackerel.

**LAMB:** Haunch, loin, fillet, or chop. Lean varieties are preferable.

**PORK:** Generally speaking, I'm not a fan of pork. Lean varieties such as fillet or meat from the Iberian pig are best. As always, quality is paramount.

**POULTRY:** Chicken, turkey, duck, goose. It is imperative to make sure that poultry is raised without hormones or antibiotics and under species-appropriate conditions. Only organic poultry should be purchased.

**SEAFOOD:** Shrimps, prawns, crab, lobster, scallops, mussels, oysters, octopus, squid, et cetera. It's often necessary to buy frozen varieties of these foods, which is by no means a bad thing.

**VEAL:** Schnitzel, fillet, haunch, and so on.

**DAIRY PRODUCTS:** Cheese, cottage cheese, curd, low-fat curd, Greek yogurt, skyr. I have included these for the sake of providing a comprehensive list. However, dairy consumption is not without its problems and is not something I recommend.

**WHEY PROTEIN:** Whey from grass-fed cattle—or, if possible, goat's (whey) protein—is highly recommended for people who do not suffer from dairy intolerance.

## Carbohydrates

Carbohydrates are the stars of the macronutrient world. We come across carbs almost on a daily basis, which are often thought of as bad foods. "Low-carb diets" seem to have become all the rage. So what's up with these carbs?

Carbohydrates are energy suppliers first and foremost. There are long- and short-chain versions of them. The spectrum of carbohydrates ranges from conventional table sugar and white flour (short-chain) to brown rice and sweet potatoes (long-chain). But what exactly is the difference? This is where biochemistry comes into play once again. The storage hormone insulin is responsible for lowering blood sugar levels. Short-chain carbohydrates, such as white table sugar, are metabolized much faster than their long-chain counterparts and therefore cause blood sugar levels to rise much faster. Insulin is then secreted in order to lower blood sugar levels again. This causes blood sugar levels to fluctuate wildly, which in turn leads to hunger pangs, and the vicious circle starts all over again. If insulin is released too often over a long period of time, this can lead to what is known as insulin resistance—where cells no longer respond to insulin stimulation—and eventually to diabetes, heart disease, and accelerated aging. Constant stimulation from insulin also leads to increased inflammation and stress in the body. If blood sugar levels drop too significantly, the stress hormone cortisol is released in order to raise blood sugars to an optimal level. This manifests as a visible increase in fat accumulation in the abdominal and hip area.

The goal of any long-term diet should be to keep blood sugars at a constant level. Long-chain carbohydrates are good for this because they take longer to digest. The more fiber a food contains, the longer this process takes and the lower the increase in blood sugars. Vegetables and fiber should be the main components of any diet because they do not require insulin to metabolize, just like healthy fats. The glycemic index indicates how significantly foods increase blood sugar levels. Foods with a high content of simple sugars or foods that are quickly converted into sugar are said to have a high glycemic index. A low glycemic index is more beneficial.

Excess carbohydrates are converted in the liver and stored as fat. Carbohydrates don't work in the same way for everyone. To be more

## What Revealing Our Stomachs Reveals About Us

Is it possible to spot if a person has a nutritional problem just from their appearance? The answer is yes. The interesting insights we have on this matter come from coaching legend Charles Poliquin. His biosignature concept uses twelve body fat measurements to determine which problems a person has, and helps them to devise a completely personalized treatment method. If fat has accumulated in the middle of the body in the form of a pot belly or "love handles," this is a sign of constantly high blood sugar and insulin levels, triggered by a diet with a high proportion of (simple) carbohydrates. This makes people more susceptible to metabolic syndrome, diabetes, heart and cardiovascular diseases, and all other forms of disease related to chronic inflammation. When a person—typically a woman—accumulates fat on their legs while the rest of the body more or less stays at a regular weight, this is a sign that a person has a problem with detoxification and excretion of toxic substances, making them prone to illnesses that stem from a hormone imbalance.

precise, the more body fat a person is carrying, the less sensitive their cells are to insulin and the less storage space the body has for sugar molecules. In a healthy body sugar is stored as glycogen in the muscle tissues. If these stores are full or have little muscle, they are instead stored as fatty tissue for any future periods of starvation. Anyone who has accumulated too much body fat around their middle should generally stay away from carbohydrates and stick to protein, vegetables, and healthy fats. This type of diet should be followed until the fat has been burned and the metabolism is working properly again. Classic paleo or low-carb high-fat diets are ideal for these people.

## GI or GL?

Unfortunately glycemic index (GI) is not precise enough to work out how different-sized portions compare. Luckily glycemic load (GL) is better suited for ranking food types.

Once the cells have been made sensitive to insulin again (as a result of a low body fat percentage), good carbohydrates should by no means be avoided, but used therapeutically (like medication) when the time is right. Ideally, they should be eaten in the evening and after training, as they favor regeneration. This is known as nutrient timing and is a method used by top athletes.

### Fruit

Fruit is generally considered to be healthy, which is true because it is rich in vitamins and antioxidants. However, in addition to glucose, it mainly contains fructose, or fruit sugar. Although fructose can be metabolized without insulin, there is only very limited storage space for fructose in the liver. Once this space becomes full, fructose is transformed into triglycerides and stored as excess fat. For healthy people one to two servings of low-glycemic fruit—for example, berries—is ideal, while people with health problems such as diabetes should avoid fruit and try to consume more vegetables and fiber. In a nutshell, those who have accumulated too much body fat are better off avoiding carbohydrates and fruit temporarily until the metabolism returns to normal. The following formula applies to weight loss:

vegetables + protein + healthy fats = healthy and slim

### Fat

During the 1990s in particular, fat was demonized. Unfortunately the fairy tale of evil fats seems to have lived on. But fat doesn't make

## Why Organic Is Not Always Best

In addition to biochemical composition, the quality of food also plays a crucial role in a healthy diet. Ultimately, we end up eating anything our food has eaten. Diet can be seen as an investment in our energy and health. Where our food comes from, how it's grown, and how good the soil is are all very important factors. Conventional methods of cultivation and husbandry use chemicals such as fertilizers, antibiotics, and hormones to increase the maximum yield of a crop or grow livestock faster. Sometimes genetics are even manipulated just to generate bigger and more profitable products. All this information is stored in the food. An organic label is not always the most helpful pointer when looking for produce of the highest quality. There are "organic" labels available for almost every food product (and even for cigarettes!). But organic labels don't really say much about foods. Where certain foods are concerned, it's better to look for a local producer who documents their production, breeding, and preservation processes and makes them transparent for consumers. Special importance should be given to species-appropriate husbandry processes. The term *organic beef* simply means that the animal has been fed with organic food, such as organic corn. However, this doesn't necessarily mean it has been well looked after. It is more important to know the farmer and be sure that they raise their cattle on pasture than to buy beef with an organic label. Beef should be 100 percent grass-fed; feeding cattle with organic grains does not change anything. It is advisable to ask the local butcher whether they have beef that is sourced in this way. If it's not possible to determine the origins of the meat, it's always better to buy organic.

## Omega-3: Megastar of the Fat World

Omega-3 fatty acids are the true stars of all fat types because they are the ultimate anti-inflammatory agents. There are three different types of omega-3 fatty acids, of which only one is considered essential because the body is not able to produce it: alpha-linolenic acid (ALA). This is mainly found in linseed oil and linseeds. The other two omega-3 fats, EPA and DHA, are not essential by definition because they can be made by the body, but it takes nine very elaborate biochemical steps to transform them. This is why it's important to absorb these valuable fatty acids directly from our diets. They can be found in fish, and especially in wild Alaskan salmon. Eicosapentaenoic acid (EPA) is the anti-inflammatory component in fish oil, while DHA (docosahexaenoic acid) is mainly responsible for cognitive ability. Our brains are made almost exclusively from fat, and in particular a fatty acid called DHA. So it's true that fish can be seen as brain food. It's thought that the human brain only started to really develop once people began eating fish—when we began settling in coastal areas. Pregnant women and children who are still growing need more DHA. Those who require high levels

us "fat," and the huge hype surrounding low-fat products has led to gross misunderstanding and ultimately, metabolic problems in many people. Excessive consumption of carbohydrates and low-fat products is partly responsible for the common diseases of today such as diabetes and heart disease. A common belief is that saturated fats are bad and adversely affect cholesterol levels. But this is not completely true. Cholesterol is the raw material required to make all sex hormones, such as estrogen and testosterone. Fats come in different varieties and have many health benefits.

of concentration on a regular basis also need more DHA, because omega-3 fatty acids make cell membranes smoother and therefore more permeable for transporting toxins out of the cell.

They have an anti-inflammatory effect and are required for any detoxification or regeneration protocol. They are also a natural blood-thinning version of aspirin or ASS (but without side effects) and increase the levels of serotonin in the brain, which means they also have an effect on our well-being. They increase the cells' sensitivity to insulin—and therefore the metabolism—and have a positive impact on blood pressure. Polyunsaturated fatty acids come in all different "flavors." Omega-6 fatty acids are mainly present in vegetable oils (rapeseed oil, sunflower oil, thistle oil) and have mainly inflammatory properties for the body. If we compare current statistics with those from 1850, however, we can see that Western diets currently contain significantly more omega-6 than omega-3 fatty acids. A high-quality omega-3 fish oil (in the form of a dietary supplement) should ideally contain EPA and DHA in a ratio of 2:1 and be free of heavy metals and other toxins.

So by no means are all saturated fats bad. Only sixty years ago per capita consumption of butter and lard was almost three times higher than it is today. There are also good alternatives to these, such as coconut oil and egg yolks. Fatty acids are the building blocks of all fats, whether in solid or liquid form. They play a crucial role in building and maintaining healthy cells. They are also a major component of cell membranes and an important energy source.

In comparison with carbohydrates or proteins, fatty acids deliver nine calories per gram, which is more than double the yield of the

## Why Margarine Is No Alternative . . . and Coconut Oil Is No Poison

Plant fats in nature only come in liquid form. Hard plant fats like margarine are created using hardening processes. *Hardened* or *part-hardened plant fats* are just synonyms for trans fats. If plant fats are overheated, trans fats are created. So keep away from fried foods (chips, fries), as well as most ready-made products (doughnuts, chocolate bars, and Nutella)! Trans fats have no place in the body, and because of their carcinogenic effects, they are already prohibited by law in most US states or must at least be labeled.

Recently coconut oil has been unjustly tarnished with a bad reputation. The plant-based fat has even been described as the "new poison." Why is this? It's true that coconut contains around 92 percent saturated fat, which we have been told is unhealthy for a long time. But we are rarely told that saturated fatty acids can be classified

former food types. Alongside saturated fats, there are also monoun-saturated and polyunsaturated fatty acids. Monounsaturated fats are found, for example, in virgin olive oil and nuts. These are not heat-stable and should not be used for frying. They are generally very good for salad dressings and can be used for steaming vegetables. They are generally very healthy and, above all, good for the heart and blood vessels. Heat-stable fats such as butter (lard), ghee, and coconut oil are more suitable for frying.

Because fats are very reactive substances and mainly react to sun and oxygen, they should always be stored in a cool, dark place. Because they also go off quickly, it's important to consume only the highest quality. The best sources can be found in organic supermarkets and health food stores. Fat doesn't make us fat; it makes us lean as either good or bad. There are saturated fatty acids that promote cardiovascular diseases and chronic inflammation, but these are mostly the trans fatty acids found in the food manufacturing industry. Unsaturated vegetable oils are chemically modified and converted to saturated fats, for example, to increase their burning point and to make them more suitable for storing. The saturated fatty acids in coconut oil are predominantly medium-chain triglycerides (MCT oils), which our bodies can rapidly convert into energy and which often have positive qualities. For example, they can help reduce the levels of bad LDL cholesterol and triglycerides in the blood, which helps prevent heart disease. They also create an environment that bad bacteria, viruses, and fungi dislike, which helps keep them at bay. Good fatty acids have another task that should not be underestimated: They are the raw material from which our bodies build the most important sex hormones.

and beautiful, if we make sure we consume good, healthy fats rather than bad ones. Fats ensure that our hormone balance is right, that cell membranes are regenerated, that skin stays nice and supple, and that our nervous system works, as well as helping to channel toxins and poisonous substances out of the body.

## Vegetables

Every individual has to find a nutrition plan that suits their constitution. Some people need more fats in their bodies, while others need more proteins. But if we can make one generalization about a type of food that everyone benefits from eating, it would of course be vegetables and plants (as always, of the best possible quality). Vegetables contain important vitamins, minerals, and neurochemicals. Because vegetables contain a lot of fiber, they are digested slowly—or to be more precise, the body burns more calories digesting them than it absorbs. Fiber slows down sugar intake and helps lower cholesterol. Vegetables hardly contain any calories, but they require more chewing and generally keep us fuller for longer. The indigestible fiber in foods in particular helps to cleanse the intestine, serves as food for the valuable microbia in the colon, and is the number one slimming agent we have access to.

Green vegetables such as broccoli, kale, and other types of cabbage contain substances that improve the body's detoxification abilities. Green vegetables, whether raw, steamed, or eaten in a salad or a smoothie, clearly come under the category of superfoods and should appear on the menu several times a day. Ideally, vegetables should account for at least 50 percent of all the food we eat.

## Food Intolerances

In all of the nutrient categories mentioned above, there are so-called superfoods and absolute no-gos: nutritional toxins. This basically means that food can be either medicine or poison. The immune system, which is supposed to be there to aggressively fight off bacteria, fungi, viruses, parasites, and other microorganisms, often ends up out of control in today's world. It simply gets confused and starts attacking everything. Food intolerances play a significant role here. The body doesn't always distinguish foreign proteins, such as gluten from wheat products or casein from dairy products, from other foreign proteins such as viruses and bacteria. Depending on how aggressive the individual immune system is, this can lead to serious, largely undetected problems. Since most conventional diets consist mainly of white flour, milk, and sugar, it's not surprising that these intolerances often develop into health problems.

## Gluten

Gluten has gained something of a celebrity status in recent years. Many people suspect they suffer from gluten intolerance, which has triggered the gluten-free trend. Gluten is a protein found in wheat, and is also known as gluten protein. It helps dough to rise in baking.

This is great for the dough, but not so great for the human organism. From a medical perspective, gluten is a powerful proinflammatory protein. It is mostly made up of two protein fractions: gluten and gliadin. Patients with celiac disease can't consume gluten, otherwise they run a significantly increased risk of developing colon cancer. Celiac disease refers to a complete intolerance to gluten, which causes people to react to the absorption of gluten with stomach cramps, diarrhea, or damage to the intestinal mucous membrane. Although this severe form of gluten intolerance affects only a small percentage of the population, many people still have a strong immune response to gluten.

Medicine has some rather strange ways of diagnosing gluten intolerance. If, for example, a one-hundred-point score were required for a celiac diagnosis, then those with a one-hundred-point score would be diagnosed, while those with ninety-nine points would not. But people in the second group nevertheless frequently suffer from problems and symptoms, which are often falsely interpreted or mistaken for other problems. If we were to try to give a precise medical definition of what counts as a gluten intolerance, all the different fractions and components of the grain and the body's reaction would have to be examined through blood tests, which would cost a considerable sum of money. It's also possible to be allergic to both the gluten and gliadin fractions. What's more, gluten is often deaminated to make it water-soluble, as it's mixed with many different products. You can even be allergic to deaminated gluten without knowing it. Lectins found in wheat and other cereals, especially the whole-grain fraction, are a problem because many people are intolerant to them. The body can also be allergic to the gluteomorphin that gluten contains. This is what makes it difficult for many people to stop eating foods with gluten in them: The stuff is just downright addictive. It can take a few days to get through the withdrawal reactions, but there are enormous health benefits to giving up gluten.

Luckily, anyone can reduce or override the overactivity of their own immune system triggered by gluten by simply avoiding it. I would advise everyone to aim toward a mainly gluten-free diet. Gluten, especially the gliadin fraction, and other substances found in the grain (lectins) can destroy the mucous membrane in

Table 4.1. Gluten-Free and Gluten-Containing
Cereals, Flours, and Starchy Foods

| Gluten-Free | Gluten-Containing |
| --- | --- |
| Amaranth | Couscous |
| Beans | Spelt |
| Bean flour (chickpeas, beans) | Einkorn |
| Buckwheat | Emmer |
| Pea flour | Flatbread |
| Garfava flour (chickpea and bean mix) | Barley |
| Gari (cassava flour) | Gluten, gluten meal |
| Gluten-free oatmeal | Graham flour |
| Millet | Semolina |
| Millet flour | Oatmeal (oat milk, flour, 98%) |
| Potato flour and starch | Durum wheat |
| Chickpeas (garbanzo beans) | Kamut |
| Linseed | Malt (malt extract, flavoring syrup, |
| Corn |   vinegar) |
| Cornmeal | Matzo flour |
| Nut flour (almond flour) | Rye |
| Arrowroot flour (maranta) | Seitan |
| Quinoa | Textured soy protein |
| Rice, all varieties | Tofu |
| Rice bran | Triticale (hybrid of wheat and rye) |
| Sago | Wheat (bran, germ, starch) |
| Tapioca (manioc, cassava, yucca) | Wheatgrass (bulgur) |
| Teff flour (dwarf millet) | Wheat flour |

the gastrointestinal tract. If this is not intact, nutrients are poorly absorbed. This leads to what is known as leaky gut syndrome (see "A Disrupted Intestinal Barrier: Leaky Gut Syndrome" on page 110). We need healthy intestinal villi to ensure maximum intake of nutritional components; otherwise we end up with vitamin, mineral, and micronutrient deficiencies. At the same time, healthy gastrointestinal mucosa is the body's barrier against unwanted invaders and contains its own immune system.

Additionally, frequent consumption of gluten causes constant inflammation in the body. Once antibodies have been formed to fight a particular virus or foreign protein such as gluten or casein, the quantity consumed no longer matters. The tiniest quantities are attacked, triggering a complete chain reaction of inflammation. In addition, chronically elevated insulin levels lead to further inflammation in the body.

Inflammatory messengers (proinflammatory cytokines) increase the body's own stress response. The body begins to produce more cortisol. Increased cortisol levels lead to an increase in the permeability of the intestinal mucosa, which in turn stimulates the immune system to release more cytokines—another classic vicious cycle.

## Dairy Products

For a long time cow's milk and dairy products have been considered healthy. Today they are among some of the biggest triggers of intolerance of all food types. In addition to triggering classic lactose intolerance, which usually causes bloating, dairy products contain many other substances that can upset the human immune system. Dairy products contain casein, a protein similar to gluten, to which many people are allergic. This type of allergy causes not an immediate reaction such as a rash or tingling and itching all over the body, but a long-term immune response induced by antibodies. The body thus forms antibodies in the same way it would to fight bacteria or viruses. This means that every time this type of food is consumed, the body will have the same immune response. And we all know the typical immune response to dietary intolerance: tiredness, fatigue, sensitivity to cold temperatures, fever, and chills in some extreme cases. In a nutshell, you're no longer as fit as you could be on a daily basis because the body is constantly busy fending off foreign substances.

One problem with the dairy products we consume today is that they are usually homogenized and pasteurized. This means they are strongly denatured using chemicals and no longer resemble cow's milk in its natural form. Raw milk usually turns sour very quickly after milking, unlike the doctored supermarket version, which is made to last for unnaturally long periods of time. A significantly higher proportion of people can tolerate raw milk in comparison to conventional milk products. Unfortunately, this is rarely available these days due to legal regulations. What's more, the conditions in which the animals are kept are often problematic. Only a small number of dairy farms nowadays are able to provide their animals with a comfortable life on pastureland, where they can eat fresh grass. Even if the majority of farmers care about the well-being of

## Butter Is Better

My aim here is not to vilify all dairy products. There are actually some that can be useful in our diets, including butter. If butter comes from grass-fed cattle that are raised exclusively on pasture, it can be classed as a superfood. Alongside healthy fats, which the body needs to build up healthy (nerve) cell membranes and hormones, it contains butyric acid, an important nutrient for gut bacteria, as well as vitamin $K_2$, a valuable vitamin for bone formation.

their animals, economic pressure and the low price of milk are forcing many to turn to intensive farming and to increase the quantities of milk they produce. The majority of these animals are fed corn and concentrated feed, and many suffer from stress as a result of the conditions in which they are raised. Of course, all of this also affects the composition and the quality of the end product. Cheap, packaged, ultra-high temperature (UHT) milk is nothing like the original milk product.

There is a lot of truth to the notion that no adult animals drink milk, and certainly not from another animal. Cow's milk is maternal milk for calves. It therefore contains all the important substances necessary for the growth of a calf, such as growth factors and hormones. As babies, we also get milk from our mothers. But this is completely different from cow's milk. The breastfeeding stage usually ends after eighteen months, and nature sees no need to switch to the milk of another animal.

Today eliminating milk from our diets is relatively easy, because there's a whole host of alternative products. For some people, it's enough to simply switch from cow's milk to sheep's or goat's milk. Otherwise, they have the option to consume unpasteurized milk (certified raw milk). There is a list of alternatives in table 4.2 for those looking to switch from animal products. Unfortunately, with the increasing range of alternatives, the list of products containing dubious ingredients is also growing. Those who opt for these alternatives should ensure that the products they buy are organically grown so that they don't contain any pesticides and haven't been genetically engineered. Sadly, soy milk and soy products are not viable alternatives as soybeans are 99 percent genetically engineered and contain so-called plant estrogens (phytoestrogen), which have no place in the human body.

## Sugar

Pure table sugar is what is known as an anti-nutrient. In addition to causing a significant impact on blood sugar levels and other associated insulin problems, sugar can only be metabolized using valuable micronutrients (vitamins, minerals, trace elements, antioxidants) in the body. Sugar is involved in the onset of diabetes, metabolic disorders, and many other chronic diseases. It should therefore be avoided.

There are no great alternatives to sugar as yet. Sweeteners such as sodium cyclamate, saccharin, or aspartame should be completely avoided because these are made purely from chemicals and their effects on the body are unpredictable. Aspartame in particular is thought to be carcinogenic. It can be found in almost all diet ("light") drinks, as well as sugar-free chewing gum and sweets. Ready-made products with bar codes and more than five ingredients should always be avoided. These products usually contain a lot of sugar, flavor enhancers, trans fats, and chemicals. If you can't read or understand the ingredients listed on the packaging, it's best to steer clear of the product. This also applies to gluten- and lactose-free products.

## Flavor Enhancers

Flavor enhancers such as glutamate—or yeast extract, as it's also known—belong to the category of dietary toxins and should always be avoided.

## Why Dietary Supplements?

Most of us do not get enough of the important vitamins and minerals we need. Some people will probably cry indignantly: "That's not true!" We are often told that we should get enough vitamins and nutrients in a normal, healthy diet. The problem is that people tend to overestimate how healthy their diets are. If you start your day with muesli, cheese spread or jam on toast, then eat meat and potatoes with gravy at lunchtime, enjoy a latte in between meals, followed by pasta or pizza for dinner (or perhaps a sandwich), this is not a healthy diet. But it is a regular diet for most people. Aside from this, the official recommended intake of vitamin C actually corresponds to the very minimum amount we need—just enough to prevent us from getting scurvy. But in times of stress or illness, or in the case of smokers, a lot more than the recommended amount of vitamin C is needed.

Of course, lifestyle plays a very important role. High stress levels, bad eating habits, smoking, alcohol, and medication all cause the body to consume more vitamins, minerals, and trace elements than is physiologically natural in order to compensate. Anyone living above the 32nd parallel north circle of latitude (which is everyone in Europe and much of the United States) also suffers a lack of sunlight and therefore of vitamin $D_3$.

Regardless of how well we feed ourselves, it's almost impossible to absorb all the necessary nutrients from today's diet. The poor quality of our soil plays an important role here. A hundred years ago a single apple had as many vitamins as 2.2 pounds of apples today. Due to overexploitation, soil quality has fallen to a minimum, and soil contains far fewer vitamins, minerals, and trace elements than we need. Unfortunately, this even applies to organic food, which is also grown on low-quality soil. Dietary supplements should by no means be considered as a form of medication, but rather as nutrition from a packet—a supplement to an ideal nutrition plan. Using supplements to make up for a bad diet is the wrong approach to take.

Dietary supplements should also be as pure as possible. This can be difficult, however, since most conventional supplements contain fillers such as magnesium stearate or silicon dioxide, dangerous dyes such as titanium oxide, anti-caking agents, and sometimes even plastics that make them resistant to gastric juices. They also often come in a capsule made from pork gelatin. It makes you wonder whether they have any health benefits at all or whether the whole thing does more harm than good. It's no wonder food supplements have a bad reputation. However, if we take food supplements that are free from all these unnecessary, partially toxic, and harmful additives—supplements that come in a plant-based capsule shell—they can be extremely useful.

## An Overview of the Most Important Nutrients

### Vitamin D$_3$

Vitamin D$_3$ is not actually a vitamin, but a hormone. It is formed in the skin as a result of solar radiation. And this is where the problem lies: We are told to avoid the sun because its rays are carcinogenic. If we have to stay out in the sun, we are told only to do so with the necessary sun protection factor. But even sun protection factor 8 reduces vitamin D$_3$ production by 97 percent.[1]

As always, dose plays a crucial role, and the dose required varies from person to person. People with darker skin need six to thirty times more sun than those with fairer skin, because they have what can be described as an "inbuilt sunscreen."[2] What's more, for optimal vitamin D$_3$ production, it's important to expose as much skin as possible to the sun. But who does this on a daily basis? When the sun is at its brightest, most people are in their offices. And what about during the winter months, when there's hardly any sun at all? Many people find themselves in chronic hibernation mode. Vitamin D$_3$ levels drop. The average levels in Germany of 30 to 60 ng/ml are very low, and by no means ideal. The body is not in a position to regenerate, repair, or rebuild itself. Only the absolute basic functions crucial to survival are maintained. It is estimated that 99 percent of people living in northern latitudes suffer from undiagnosed vitamin D$_3$ deficiency. Recommendations are constantly being shifted to higher values.

Just a few years ago, the recommended daily intake for vitamin D$_3$ was 600 IU (international units). This has now been raised to 2,000 IU per day. From experience, I would say the dose should be more like 5,000 to 10,000 IU per day. Need for vitamin D$_3$, however, increases immensely if there are chronic stressors in the body, as well as after surgery.[3]

Vitamin $D_3$ is crucial for almost every process in the body. Over the last few years, it has been discovered that every cell in the body has vitamin $D_3$ receptors. It helps the immune system to regulate itself better. It can be thought of as a kind of brake for the modern immune system's overactivity. It helps with all kinds of colds, flus, and allergies in which the immune system plays a role. Vitamin $D_3$ is the key to healthy bone and tooth mineralization and is therefore always included in my treatments. Several studies show that vitamin D deficiency leads to problems in bone and tooth development, gastrointestinal and neurological problems such as multiple sclerosis, ADD, depression, schizophrenia, and even cancers.[4]

Supplements should aim to provide a quantity of vitamin $D_3$ somewhere in the mid- to high range of the recommended dose. High doses of vitamin $D_3$ should always be medically monitored and never taken without the important co-factors. Nutrients always work as a team in the body (synergistically), unlike medication, which usually floods or blocks specific areas. This works a bit like a soccer team. If a team were made up only of strikers, it would be impossible to win a game. If vitamin $D_3$ is the striker, then vitamin $K_2$ is the goalkeeper and zinc and magnesium are right and left midfielders. It's important to have all players on board—and if possible a couple of extras on the bench.

**Magnesium**

Magnesium deficiency is very widespread. It's mostly associated with calf muscle cramps, but magnesium is actually involved in over three hundred metabolic processes. It's the ultimate relaxation mineral and helps with headaches, migraines, muscle tension, and cramps. Magnesium, together with vitamin $K_2$ and zinc, plays a prominent role in bone metabolism and tissue building, and is required for the activation of vitamin $D_3$.[5] It's involved in almost all detoxification processes and is responsible for keeping the heart rate regular. Magnesium is also a co-factor in blood sugar regulation and improves the cells' sensitivity to insulin. It's consumed extremely quickly by stress. Finally, it helps improve sleep quality, thanks to its relaxing properties. Magnesium is found mainly in dark, leafy vegetables, nuts, seeds, fish, meat, and avocados.

## Zinc

Zinc deficiency is also among the most common nutrient deficiencies. Like magnesium, zinc is involved as a co-factor in over three hundred different metabolic processes in the body. Zinc improves wound healing processes and is therefore often used in creams. It should also be used in all postoperative nutrient protocols. It can help with skin problems such as eczema, dry skin, general wound healing disorders, and acne. The same applies to our mucous membranes. Whenever signs of inflammation such as bleeding gums or intestinal mucosal inflammations such as ulcerative colitis or Crohn's disease appear, zinc should be the first port of call. Together with vitamin $D_3$, vitamin $K_2$, and magnesium, it plays a key role in bone metabolism and is also involved as a co-factor of numerous enzymes in the detoxification cycle. Like magnesium, zinc plays an important role in maintaining balanced sugar levels and improves the cells' insulin sensitivity levels. Zinc is also known for its immunomodulatory properties. Like vitamin $D_3$, it can be thought of as a brake that helps the immune system to regulate itself better. Zinc stimulates the growth of white blood cells and is involved in the production of the hormone thymulin. It is also involved in the production of sex hormones and has been proven to increase testosterone, and therefore libido. It blocks aromatase, an enzyme that increases the conversion rate of testosterone to estrogen, which is especially important in men. Sperm—and therefore fertility—also benefit from zinc intake. Both magnesium and zinc should always come together in an organic compound known as a chelate. Magnesium citrate / glycinate / malate / gluconate are highly recommended.

## Vitamin C

We all know vitamin C as the ultimate super vitamin. Whenever we have a cold, we reach for vitamin C. It can be found in many fruits or in the supermarket as pure ascorbic acid. Since this form of the vitamin is highly acidic and therefore incompatible with teeth and gastric mucosa, I recommend taking a buffered version. There is still a misconception that oranges contain high quantities of vitamin C, and some companies take advantage of this in their advertising. The foods with the highest vitamin C quantities are raw beetroot and rose hips. Orange juice, on the other hand, is like a lemonade that makes adults think they are being healthy—but ultimately it's just another sugary drink. The recommended daily allowance of vitamin C is calculated to prevent people from getting scurvy, a horrible maritime disease that causes people to lose all their teeth. It's indispensable for tissue building and should be taken immediately for wound healing disorders or when signs of inflammation occur, such as bleeding gums. Of course, vitamin C also plays a crucial role in strengthening the immune system, has antibacterial and antiviral properties, and is one of the main antioxidants in the body. Oxidation is constantly caused by free radicals in the body, which antioxidants can help to catch. We see this process happen frequently in apples. Oxidation takes place when we leave a slice of apple out in the air for a while. Within just a short time, the fruit begins to turn brown. This also happens in our bodies with cells that are particularly susceptible to the oxidation process. Vitamin C is an anti-stress vitamin and is crucial for the production and regeneration of adrenal hormones and messengers such as cortisol and adrenaline.

The vitamin C requirement is higher for those suffering from diseases and stress, as well as smokers, athletes, and anyone who has just had an operation. One cigarette uses up the basic daily requirement of vitamin C. Just imagine what happens if a person smokes half a pack per day, is stressed at work, and happens to have a cold. The daily requirement for vitamin C is regulated by our stool. Too much vitamin C is simply excreted by the body. I generally recommend taking 2 to 3 grams of vitamin C per day, if possible in an easy-to-process, buffered form. Before, during, and after surgical procedures in the mouth area, high doses of vitamin C infusions have been proven to be very beneficial in preventing infections.

## Foods for a Healthy Bacterial Flora

If the bacterial flora in the mouth and gut are healthy, this contributes greatly to the body's immune system. Probiotic foods—foods that are good for a healthy microbial flora—improve the defense mechanisms of the epithelium in the gastrointestinal tract and help with the utilization of nutrients and energy. The healthier the mouth and the oral microbia are, the healthier the digestive tract, immune system, and body are as a whole. Unhealthy and especially sweet foods are unfortunately not only appetizing to us, but also favorites of the bad bacteria in the mouth and intestine. If we feed ourselves these foods, we also feed these bacteria and help them to grow.

Sugar and other simple carbohydrates, such as those we eat today in large quantities, are not normally found in nature. When we do eat these foods in nature, first they grow in such a way that we have to work to be able to consume them, and second they support the growth of healthy bacteria. This is because in nature, sugar only comes in its natural shell. When humans or animals want to get to carbohydrates, they usually have to break up this shell of plant fibers first. This shell provides the microbes in the mouth and intestine with fibers that help to form a balanced microbial environment. Now, however, industrialization has given us access to white refined sugar and ground white flour. These are the main culprits that upset the microbia. Our bodies and teeth are the ones that have to suffer the consequences.[6] The shells in which carbohydrates are usually found contain fibers that promote what is known as the anti-obesity effect. This means they help to reduce our weight and break down fat, as well as being anti-inflammatory.

If we regularly only eat macronutrients from protein, carbohydrates, and fat without eating enough vegetables, the microbia in the large intestine starve because these nutrients are all absorbed by the small intestine. The only option our cohabitants occupying the large intestine have is to eat the mucous membrane, which of course leads to inflammation in the body. Many of the fibers in our diet, especially the insoluble types (also known as prebiotics), however, provide the perfect snack for our friends in the large intestine, and as an added bonus, they also metabolize short-chain fatty acids (SCFAs), providing us with energy directly. Now, that's a win-win situation.

Probiotics, which are good for a healthy intestinal flora, are found mainly in fermented dishes such as sauerkraut, kimchi, and gherkins. These are of great value as a dietary supplement, especially for anyone who has ever taken antibiotics, and are particularly useful just after a course of antibiotics. Good supplements contain at least four to six types of different strains of probiotics in large quantities (one to forty billion per unit).

Prebiotics are indigestible fibers. These are anti-inflammatory, improve mineral absorption, and serve as food for our intestinal bacteria. As described above, the intestinal bacteria from insoluble fiber produce an important energy source for us: SCFAs. They occur naturally in a large variety of plants, such as garlic, chicory, artichokes, onions, and asparagus.

Ideally we should aim to consume a minimum of 10 to 20 grams of these each day. Some good sources include psyllium husks, guar gum, and FOS (fructooligosaccharides). A supplement that contains both pre- and probiotics is therefore the ideal solution.

## Case Study: How Food Affects Our Mood

Our intestines are home to our immune systems and are also where food is digested and important nutrients from our food filtered out. But the influence of the intestine on our mood, feelings, and behavior remains largely overlooked. We primarily connect emotions with the mind or heart, but in reality many come from the stomach. "Go with your gut!" people often tell us. In fact, this advice is not necessary, because we do it all the time whether we like it or not. But how can the gut influence our mood?

What many people don't know is that most of the body's neurotransmitters are found in the gut, which is why it's sometimes referred to as our second brain. Our main neurotransmitters are called dopamine, acetylcholine, GABA, and serotonin. Neurotransmitters are messenger substances similar to hormones that the body requires to transmit stimuli and information. They are responsible for biochemically forwarding electrical information from the nervous system to the receptors of the subsequent target cells. At the end of the day, neurotransmitters determine who we are, how we feel, how we behave, and what decisions we make.

A shortage of neurotransmitters may determine many of our actions, because we unconsciously act to compensate for deficiencies. Unfortunately, these compensation strategies are not always

## A True Test

Ninety-five percent of neurotransmitters are formed in the gastrointestinal tract, but only 5 percent of them make it to the brain—and these are the ones that count. Stools are often examined to measure the balance of neurotransmitters in the body. But the 5 percent that arrive in the brain are much more interesting. If you want to get to know your neurotransmitter profile, all you have to do is fill in a questionnaire designed by US psychologist Eric Braverman. Take the questionnaire online here: https://www.bravermantest.com.

good for us. If we have a sudden craving for greasy chips, for example, this might not just indicate a lack of discipline. It could also be a—rather unhealthy—strategy we use for quick stimulation. Poor nutrition can therefore lead to neurotransmitter deficiencies, but a neurotransmitter deficiency can also lead to poor nutrition. Another vicious circle.

It's therefore best not to get into this negative spiral in the first place and to slip into a state of deficiency. It's possible to ensure we eat foods that promote the formation of neurotransmitters, which in turn will have an impact on mood, sleep quality, and motivation.

The most important raw materials our body uses to make neurotransmitters are amino acids, which are the smallest components of proteins. For many people, a lack of protein alone is responsible for a lack of neurotransmitters—they simply lack the raw materials they need for their bodies to form these messenger substances. Again, certain co-factors play an important role here, such as activated B vitamins, magnesium, and the omega-3 fatty acids mentioned above, which support the formation of neurotransmitters. Anyone who wants to feel good and enjoy life should make sure their gut is happy. If inflammatory processes take place there, this also impairs the formation of neurotransmitters, which is enough in itself to trigger mental health issues.

## Dopamine

The most important messenger for energy is dopamine, which is also known as the motivation molecule. Dopamine deficiency can manifest in depression-like symptoms: a lack of motivation, tiredness, fatigue, addiction, procrastination, sleeping problems, low libido, moodiness, aggression, and difficulty concentrating. Put simply: Our lust for life disappears.

Foods that stimulate dopamine production include red meat (beef, lamb, veal), chicken, eggs, sardines, and salmon. Other nutrients such as B vitamins, chlorella, omega-3, vitamin C, and activated (methylated) folic acid (found in green leafy vegetables and chlorella) also help dopamine kick into action.

## Acetylcholine

Another important neurotransmitter is acetylcholine. This is the messenger for creativity, impulsiveness, intuition, and innovation—it makes us sociable and charismatic, motivates us and sparks our thirst for adventure. If we don't have enough of it, we start to notice memory loss, language difficulties, learning difficulties, and an overall loss of enthusiasm.

Foods that promote the formation of acetylcholine include healthy fats made from butter, nuts, salmon, egg yolk, and meat. But

### Useless Tricks

Some people unconsciously engage in unhealthy dopamine self-medication by frequently consuming sugar, caffeine, or nicotine, but these substances are just a quick fix and never last as long as a proper boost.

instead many people get a quick hit from fatty foods such as chips and chocolate.

## GABA

GABA can be described as nature's Valium. It ensures emotional and mental stability and provides the impulse that makes us care for others. Those with a GABA deficiency are not able to shut down easily, get stressed quickly, have chaotic thoughts before falling asleep, and/or are susceptible to anxiety, panic attacks, and irritable bowel syndrome.

Foods that stimulate GABA include healthy carbohydrates (in the evening), lentils, protein, and in particular an amino acid called glutamine.

## Serotonin

Perhaps the most well-known neurotransmitter is serotonin. This is the molecule that keeps us happy and satisfied. A lack of serotonin often manifests in depression, anxiety, low self-esteem, eating disorders, and insomnia. A large proportion of serotonin is made from one of the building blocks in the gut known as tryptophan. Foods rich in tryptophan include healthy carbohydrates as well as protein from turkey, mackerel, white meat, and fish. A serotonin deficiency is often the cause for cravings for sweets, pasta, pizza, or rice, but it should of course be satisfied with healthy foods instead.

## How to Approach Your New Nutrition Plan

It should be easy for anyone to build their own individual nutrition plan with the aid of figure 4.1, table 4.1, table 4.2, and table 4.3. Your individual nutrition plan should be based on your current state of health and what goals you want to achieve for yourself (see "Individual Goals and Recommendations" later in this chapter).

I generally recommend the Life Changer plan to all of my patients for the first fourteen days, because it helps the body switch from metabolizing sugar to metabolizing fat. I call it this because people quickly feel that something is changing when they follow the program. For a minimum period of fourteen days, all foods from the "Allergy

Triggers, Toxins" column of table 4.2 (page 157) as well as the "Gluten-Containing" column of table 4.1 (page 142) are completely off-limits to eliminate all food intolerances, toxins, and inflammatory factors. This regulates blood sugar levels, improves inflammation in the gastrointestinal tract, and generally reduces the body's tendency toward inflammation. This first step might also be called the elimination phase. The body is finally able to rest and is given "real food" that it can use to build up tissue and the neurotransmitters mentioned above. After this initial period, and depending on your goal and how good you feel, it's also possible to switch to either the 90:10 or the 80:20 plan.

**What Is 80:20?**
The expression *80:20* refers to getting 80 percent of food from the "Superfoods" category, and 10 percent (one portion per day) from

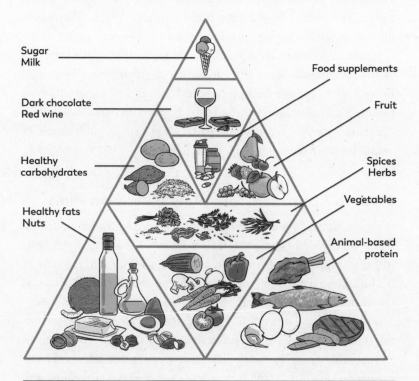

**Figure 4.1.** The ideal food pyramid.

Table 4.2. Allergy Triggers, Toxins, and Their Alternatives

| Type | Allergy Triggers, Toxins | Alternatives |
|---|---|---|
| Dairy | Yogurt<br>Milk<br>Curd<br>Cheese | Plant-based:<br>• Coconut milk and yogurt<br>• Almond milk and yogurt<br>• Cashew milk and yogurt<br>• Hazelnut milk<br><br>Animal-based:<br>• Goat's milk and yogurt<br>• Sheep's milk and yogurt |
| Sugar | Glucose-free syrup<br>Fructose (in large quantities) found in dried fruit, juices, and sugary drinks, sandwich spreads and Nutella, agave syrup and milk chocolate<br>Found in diet products, chewing gum, sweets, and soft drinks | Honey (organic)<br>Maple syrup<br>Dark chocolate with a cocoa component over 70<br>Ice cream (coconut-based) |
| Sweeteners | Acesulfame K<br>Aspartame<br>Cyclamate<br>Saccharin<br>Sucralose<br>Found in diet products, chewing gum, sweets, and soft drinks | Xylitol (birch sugar)<br>Erythritol<br>Stevia |
| Stimulants | Glutamate<br>Aspartame<br>Nicotine | Coffee, 1 to 2 cups per day (organic), depending on individual tolerance levels |
| Flavor Enhancers | Glutamate<br>Yeast extract<br>Found in instant noodles, soy sauce, stock cubes, ready meals and sauces | Gluten-free soy sauce (tamari)<br>Organic vegetable broth without flavor enhancers |
| Trans Fats | Hardened vegetable fat<br>Found in margarine, fried foods, chips, Nutella, and ready-made sauces | No alternatives! |
| Other | Known allergens<br>Ready-made meals<br>Soy products<br>Rule of thumb: Foods that contain more than five ingredients you can't pronounce should generally be avoided.<br>Alcohol: Depends on the amount. Enjoy in moderation. A glass of dry red wine contains important antioxidants. | No alternatives! |

*Note:* For foods containing gluten and gluten-free alternatives, see table 4.1.

Table 4.3. Superfoods

| Protein | Good Carbohydrates | Healthy Fats | Fruit | Vegetables |
|---|---|---|---|---|
| Lean meat:<br>• Pasture-fed beef<br>• Lamb<br>• Veal<br>• Game<br><br>Free-range poultry:<br>• Chicken<br>• Turkey<br><br>Fish and seafood:<br>• Oysters<br>• Trout<br>• Cod<br>• Alaskan salmon<br>• Mackerel<br>• Octopus<br>• Sardines<br>• Shrimps, prawns<br>• Pike perch<br><br>Plant-based:<br>• Quinoa<br>• Chlorella<br>• Legumes | Amaranth<br>Buckwheat<br>Gari<br>Gluten-free grains (see table 4.1)<br>Pumpkin<br>Manioc<br>Quinoa<br>Rice:<br>• Basmati<br>• Jasmine<br>• Plain<br>Sweet potato<br>Potato<br>Vegetables | Avocado<br>Butter<br>Lard<br>Egg yolk<br>Ghee<br>Hemp oil<br>Coconut milk<br>Coconut oil<br>Linseed oil<br>Nut oils (e.g. walnut oil)<br>Olive oil (virgin)<br>Omega-3 fish oil<br>Seeds and kernels:<br>• Hemp seeds<br>• Hazelnuts<br>• Macadamia nuts<br>• Almonds<br>• Brazil nuts<br>• Pecan nuts<br>• Pine nuts<br>• Pistachios<br>• Walnuts<br>• Nut spreads or butters | Açai<br>Pineapple<br>Apple<br>Apricot<br>Bananas<br>Blueberries<br>Dates<br>Strawberries<br>Figs<br>Grapefruit<br>Raspberries<br>Honeydew<br>Cherries<br>Kiwi<br>Mandarin<br>Mango<br>Cantaloupe<br>Oranges<br>Pear<br>Plums<br>Grapes | Artichoke<br>Cauliflower<br>Broccoli<br>Fennel<br>Kale<br>Cucumber<br>Carrots<br>Cabbage<br>Leek<br>Chard<br>Eggplant<br>Paprika<br>Parsnip<br>Mushrooms<br>Brussels sprouts<br>Beetroot<br>Salad<br>Sauerkraut<br>Asparagus<br>Spinach<br>Tomato<br>Zucchini<br>Onion |

*Note:* Of course, it's impossible to provide an exhaustive list in one table. This list is simply intended as a compass to point people in the right direction toward a healthier lifestyle.

the "Good Carbohydrates" category, ideally in the evening or after exercise rather than for breakfast, and the remaining 10 percent from the "Allergy Triggers, Toxins, and Their Alternatives" category. This means sticking to roughly one portion of carbohydrates, ideally consumed around exercise (preferably after) or in the evening (to make the most of the relaxing effect of carbohydrates).

## Individual Goals and Recommendations

**GOAL:** *I'm a competitive sportsperson and need to optimize my performance.*

**RECOMMENDATION:** Eat 100 percent superfoods, including the intelligent consumption of good carbohydrates as well as foods like bananas that are easy to digest straight after exercise to replenish glycogen stores. The meal after exercise at least should contain a portion of sweet potatoes or rice (good carbohydrates). It makes sense to compose meals from macronutrients, protein, and good carbohydrates, as fats would be a hindrance to digestion at this time. Unlimited amounts of vegetables can be eaten at any time. It's advisable to combine pre-exercise meals with macronutrients, protein, healthy fats and vegetables to boost energy for the upcoming training session to the maximum and to increase neurotransmitters dopamine and acetylcholine for the working day.

**GOAL:** *I'm satisfied, but would like to feel even better.*

**RECOMMENDATION:** Follow the fourteen-day Life Changer, followed by the 80:20 program. Depending on insulin sensitivity (body fat percentage), add one portion of good carbohydrates in the evening.

**GOAL:** *I'm chronically ill and want to get my health back.*

**RECOMMENDATION:** Eat 100 percent superfoods. It's difficult to recommend a one-size-fits-all diet in the case of chronic diseases. The utmost priority is, however, to avoid all foods that could in any way stress the immune, digestive, or nervous system (table 4.2). Depending on the clinical picture, a ketogenic and vegan diet should be followed for a certain period of time to rule out any growth and inflammatory factors. It may also be necessary to heavily control the intake of free amino acids to ensure that the body is not deficient in any of these. In these cases it's important to talk to an experienced doctor, dentist, alternative practitioner, or other coach/therapist.

**GOAL:** *I have a few health problems I would like to get rid of.*

**RECOMMENDATION:** Follow the fourteen-day Life Changer, followed by the 80:20 or 90:10 program, depending on the level of improvement seen. The aim must always be to relieve the burden on the digestive and nervous systems as much as possible.

---

For some people, this requires some discipline in the beginning. But because it's possible to feel the positive effects very quickly, often people don't want to return to their old diets, especially because they realize that they start to feel worse when they fall back into the habit of eating unhealthy foods. Generally I recommend a diet similar to the paleo diet to everyone—one that releases little to no insulin. Carbohydrates are mostly beneficial for those who do a lot of sports and have low body fat percentages. For everyone else, they shouldn't appear on the menu as often. To put it another way, carbs have to be earned.

However, it's always better for the body to switch from the usual carbohydrate sources, such as sugar and white flour, to healthy carbohydrates from table 4.3.

The best way to keep our diets simple and healthy is to imagine that we are still hunter-gatherers—albeit smartphone-wielding, headphone-wearing hunter-gatherers. Even though there is a virtually infinite choice of foods to choose from today, our genetics have not changed in the last ten thousand years and we need to remember what we ate when there were no chemicals or ready-made products. We should therefore primarily choose foods that we could theoretically hunt, fish, or gather.

## Keeping Your Teeth Healthy

### Dental Care for Children

Dental hygiene is important from the very beginning of our lives. For many children, however, it starts a bit too early. Often new parents are given special tablets, which they are told to give their newborn babies every day from then on. The tablets are made from a mixture of vitamin D and fluoride. I am convinced that it's a good thing to give people—including children—vitamin D and personally recommend it, but it should be taken on its own rather than in combination with fluoride. I have explained my critical stance on fluoride (see "Fluoride: The Best Means of Fighting Tooth Decay?" on page 21), and feel even more strongly about it for children.

Parents are not generally told that dentists' and pediatricians' views on fluoride vary. While the German Society for Dental and Oral Medicine does not recommend fluoride, stating that brushing with fluoridated toothpaste as soon as a child gets their first tooth is sufficient, pediatricians recommend standardized administration of fluoride, despite the fact that it's been proven that fluoride is most effective when applied locally. Why we should burden a very young, developing organism with fluoride for years on end is beyond me. Many parents give their children fluoride tablets as well as fluoridated toothpaste simply because they don't know any better. This, added to the fluoride found in food and drink, can push intake levels up to levels that can result in an overdose. This sometimes manifests in the form of "fluorosis"—whitish discolorations that appear on the teeth, which can also turn yellow or brown. At an advanced stage, fluorosis makes teeth significantly more sensitive.

Many pediatricians deny that there is a link between fluoride tablets and the symptoms parents see in their children. Skeptics will often say: "This has been working for decades." But this is not a valid argument because the side effects and illnesses that often only appear years later are not put into context.

Those who want their children to have healthy teeth and growth would do better to ensure that their children are eating the right diet with enough nutrients. Brushing teeth as soon as the first tooth comes through and avoiding sticky sweets and snacks are certainly far better than years of taking a controversial chemical.

## Dental Care in Later Life

Until not so long ago, it almost seemed to be considered a law of nature: As you get older, you lose your teeth. It was seen as normal to expect to have one's "third set of teeth" at some point in life. As recently as 1997 every fourth person between the age of sixty-five and seventy-four no longer had any of their own teeth. Today the figure stands at every eighth.[7] A recent study shows how strong the correlation between dental hygiene and overall health is. Researchers at Boston University and Columbia University have found that people over the age of seventy-four have a much greater chance of living long lives if they still have a full set of teeth.

Furthermore, the results show that participants who have already lost five or more teeth by the age of sixty-five are at a higher risk for health problems such as heart disease or diabetes. The study clearly confirms the basic assumption of biological dentistry: If a person loses their teeth, this can be a clear sign of other diseases that reduce life expectancy. Since oral health is a reliable indicator of general health, it's important to always pay special attention to it.[8]

So good oral health is something we should definitely strive for into old age—and this is very easy to do. Nutrition and nutrient supply are the most important factors. The older a person is, the more likely they are to have nutrient deficiencies. Older people often suffer from a lack of vitamin $D_3$ and should have their levels checked regularly. I generally recommend maintaining a vitamin $D_3$ value of above 50 ng/ml, and ideally over 70 ng/ml before surgery. From the age of around sixty, the production of vitamin $D_3$ in the body decreases, which means it's crucial to take supplements.

A common problem for older people from a dentist's perspective is what is known as root caries. Because the gums begin to recede in older age, the tooth neck becomes exposed, making teeth particularly susceptible to decay. If gum retraction is accompanied by aggressive brushing, crowns can also show signs of aging and become porous. Tooth neck decay is made worse by a lack of saliva in the mouth. Saliva production decreases with age, but many medicines taken by older people also cause dry mouth as a side effect. Drinking and chewing a lot is very important because this stimulates the flow of saliva.

Often two factors coincide unfavorably when we get to a certain age. On the one hand patients have more restorative dentures such as implants, bridges, and crowns in the mouth, and on the other patients' motor skills decline, making them unable to give their teeth the necessary care and cleaning. This is why older people should have their teeth professionally cleaned more than twice a year if possible.

Special care should be taken with removable dentures. Prostheses can be breeding grounds for bacteria and cause dangerous infections because bacteria, fungi, and other pathogens can settle and multiply both under and on prostheses. In 2015 Japanese researchers found that seniors who leave their removable dentures in their mouth overnight are twice as likely to suffer from pneumonia as those who remove their dentures to sleep. This presents a dilemma because wearing dentures at night can prevent the jawbone from regressing. What's more, certain patients find it easier to get used to their dentures if they are worn at night. The German Society for Pneumology and Respiratory Medicine also points out the risks of sleeping with dentures in, citing results of recent studies.

There is nothing wrong with wearing full dentures as long as they are well made and the patient does not have any adverse reactions to them and is able to clean them properly. In general, however, people can be given fixed dentures. Removable prostheses are used less and less and will soon probably only be seen in museums.

## Staying Healthy: FAQs About Dental Care

Obviously it's best to keep your own teeth for as long as possible. The right diet is the most important factor here. But of course dental hygiene also plays a big role. Given that there is still a lot of uncertainty surrounding this topic, I've put together some of the most frequently asked questions along with my answers.

*After eating, or once in the morning and once in the evening: How often should you brush your teeth?*
Personally, I brush my teeth once a day in the morning. I have never had a cavity and I don't believe I would get one even if I stopped brushing my teeth in the morning. But that's because my diet matches the nutrition plan described above almost 100 percent. I rarely eat carbohydrates and very rarely touch sugar, plus I make sure I regularly get additional nutrients. I am convinced that this is a more important factor for avoiding tooth decay than regular dental hygiene. However, this should not be understood as a recommendation to let

good oral hygiene slip. For those who can't manage eating healthily all the time, I recommend the classic cleaning routine in the morning and at night.

### What's the best type of toothbrush to use?

I always recommend using an ultrasonic toothbrush. If used correctly, it can leave your teeth very clean. Those who prefer to brush manually can continue to do so, but electric toothbrushes are generally always better than manual. However, the same principle applies to both methods: Always brush in a circular motion without applying too much pressure, and never scrub.

### Which toothpaste is the best?

In my opinion, the perfect toothpaste hasn't been invented yet. Most products are full of dubious additives that have no place in the mouth—including the fluoride mentioned earlier, but also many other problematic additives, including a harmful substance called titanium oxide (a white coloring also known as E171). I always recommend fluoride-free toothpaste to my patients, preferably with an aloe vera base. In addition, toothpaste shouldn't contain any abrasive particles that could damage the enamel. These are typically found in toothpastes that are supposed to whiten teeth. Stay clear of these.

### Does mouthwash improve oral hygiene?

Mouthwash solutions promise to freshen breath, destroy bacteria, and soothe inflamed gums—and I think they are all unnecessary. Some chemical rinses even have a negative effect: They are harmful to the mouth and the periodontium because they disturb and disrupt the oral flora. If you want to do something good for your teeth aside from just brushing them, you should pull oil instead. Fish oil would be a very healthy oil for doing this—but admittedly it isn't for the fainthearted. Virgin coconut, walnut, almond, and olive oil are much more pleasant. Coconut oil has the added benefit of being antibacterial and antiviral. Oil pulling is very easy to do. Keep a tablespoon of oil in your mouth for as long as possible, and after a minimum of five minutes, spit it out again—don't swallow.

*Should I have my teeth professionally cleaned on a regular basis?*
That's something I definitely recommend, yes! You should have your teeth professionally cleaned at least twice a year. Anyone with implants, bridges, and/or crowns should have their teeth cleaned even more frequently. This is because it's impossible to clean as thoroughly as a trained specialist by yourself. Professional dental cleaning should not be a chore—I see it as a kind of cosmetic treatment. Afterward, teeth are polished white and pleasantly smooth.

*What else can help whiten teeth?*
I recommend what is known as an in-house bleaching to anyone who wants whiter teeth. This takes place in a dentist's practice after a professional cleaning. It lasts an hour to an hour and a half and leaves you with visibly whiter teeth after just one session. The downside is that sometimes teeth are sensitive for a while afterward. Another version of this treatment is having impressions of your teeth taken after a professional cleaning, which are then used to create bleaching rails. These can be brushed with a whitening agent and worn at home, for example at night. It takes around two weeks to reach the desired result. The advantage is that you can rebleach your teeth whenever you feel like it without having to go to the dentist's. The downside is that teeth react sensitively to red wine, coffee, and green tea during the treatment period, which is why it should be used sparingly. It's also important to make sure that only natural tooth substance is whitened as opposed to crowns or fillings, so there can sometimes be differences between fillings and teeth after bleaching. If carried out incorrectly, bleaching can therefore damage the enamel and is therefore best left in professional hands. It's best to steer clear of home remedies such as baking soda with lemon or whitening strips.

*I have sensitive teeth. What can I do about it?*
One product you can use for sensitive teeth is tooth mousse, a fluoride-free paste low in chemicals with mineral components. However, it can be difficult to apply. In any case, it's better to solve the problem through nutrition. Sensitive teeth are a sign of mineral and micronutrient deficiencies, especially vitamin $D_3$.

*I have implants and bridges. Is regular brushing enough to
maintain them?*
Any type of dentures require a bit more care than regular teeth. The
most important thing to remember is to have your teeth professionally cleaned more than twice a year.

*I don't just want to have my teeth repaired, and my overall health is
important to me. Which type of dentist should I see?*
Conventional dentistry still pays too little attention to the overall
health of patients. This is why I currently only recommend dentists
who are specially trained in biological dentistry. These dentists always
think of the organism as a whole when devising a treatment approach.

*But isn't all this very expensive?*
Most services offered in biological dentistry are not covered by health
insurance so patients have to pay for them. Investing money in our
health, and especially in the prevention of illnesses, is difficult for
many people. Yet we are almost all willing to spend money if we are ill
and have a chance of recovering. Sometimes we have to decide what
to spend money on: the next holiday, an expensive smartphone, or
our health. If health is your number one priority, you can always find
a way. People who are struggling financially can also start gradually:
First have all the metals removed from your mouth, which often
brings great relief to the whole body.

*I'm really terrified of going to the dentist.*
Dentists work in a very delicate and sensitive area. But today we have the
option to make any treatment virtually painless. Since I started working
as a biological dentist, all of my patients look forward to their appointments because they know they will finally be able to get to the bottom of
their problems and find a solution (which they have sometimes waited
a long time for). The focus is clearly on health. In the future I would
very much like all patients to be happy to visit the dentist, knowing that
we can help them to improve or regain their health.

# The Case for a New Dentistry

*First they ignore you,*
*then they laugh at you,*
*then they fight you,*
*then you win.*

—Mahatma Gandhi

Medicine is changing. A theory is only ever valid until it can be replaced with an alternative. But sometimes this takes a very long time, because the old paradigms in our minds and textbooks live on beyond their sell-by date. Certain medical breakthroughs are so revolutionary that they dramatically shape the way diseases are perceived and treated for decades. One such change was the discovery of penicillin almost a hundred years ago. The advent of antibiotics has not only saved lives but also decisively shaped the patterns in the way we look at and treat diseases to this day. To put it simply, the pattern goes something like this:

- The patient's disease has a concrete cause.
- The doctor prescribes a drug that fights this specific cause alone.
- The patient gets better.

If something works well and successfully, people want to repeat it. We could say that medicine and science today are still influenced by the patterns that provided the basis for the antibiotic revolution. Doctors try to treat illnesses mainly by prescribing medication. At the same time, medical science is pursuing the hopeful credo of finally achieving a breakthrough against suffering. But today we are fighting against different illnesses than the ones we saw a hundred years ago. These modern illnesses don't usually have just one cause that we can take medication for. The causes are often diverse, specific to the individual, and usually only discoverable when we look at the history and lifestyle of a patient.

Conventional medicine still turns to the old paradigms for diseases of the twenty-first century, sometimes because the health care system doesn't allow for anything else. On average, a doctor has just less than seven minutes to see each patient. Ninety percent of appointments are spent talking about symptoms and related medications. Medicine today has standard treatments for diseases with different causes. The focus is always on the disease, rather than the person's health. Rarely does medicine offer tailor-made solutions—though there are some. Most illnesses people are suffering from today did not simply break out like an infection. They are mostly acquired as a result of our modern lifestyles. This is why we also need other, new ways of dealing with them.

It might seem an unusual choice to start this process in the mouth—some people even laugh at the thought or try to downplay the importance of oral hygiene. But dentistry is changing, too. It has done valuable and considerable work as a repair medicine. Whereas not so long ago, the only possible treatment was tooth extraction, today there are other options available that are not only tolerable but also aesthetically perfect. Although we now know a lot more about techniques, materials, and the right precautions to take, in terms of pure detail work, modern dentistry is restricted primarily to its traditional working environment: the mouth. Modern dentistry can and should look far beyond this area. A new dentistry should broaden its focus to involve the rest of the body. Research has already clearly shown us the way: The connections between disease in the mouth and chronic disease elsewhere in the body are unambiguous, and gradually new theories are paving the way in our minds and textbooks.

Biological dentistry does not aim to act as a supplement or alternative to traditional dentistry, but as an extension. It's about jumping over holes rather than digging them deeper. It aims to bring disciplines together rather than disrupt them. I dream of a world where dentistry and general medicine do not form separate spheres, but work hand in hand. I dream of a medicine that rejects the idea of separating the body into sections and instead acquires more knowledge about integrative concepts. I dream of a medicine that trains both patients and doctors to understand our organism as a whole. A medicine that understands what causes disruption, but also how the body can regenerate and heal. A progressive form of medicine, oriented toward health issues people are facing today, needs to do more than dole out diagnoses and treatments. It should give people all the information and tools they need to integrate health concepts into their daily lives so that they can take their life and health into their own hands instead of fatefully having to accept illnesses. I am firmly convinced that this is the right way to respond to the medical challenges of the twenty-first century—and if need be, this path will be led by dentistry. This may sound unimaginable today, but tomorrow we might just start getting used to the idea. In the not-too-distant future, my hope is that this way of thinking will become completely normal.

Let the healing begin!

# ACKNOWLEDGMENTS

First of all, I'd like to thank the people who have helped me on my personal journey. This list doesn't follow any particular order—I'm simply following my heart. Thank you Mum and Dad, for always supporting me and continuing to support me, even though I'm sure I've been a challenge at times. Thank you to my little bro and best friend Flo, who still looks after me and wants to change the world with me. Thank you to my little sister Lulu, for always believing in me. Thank you to my friends Big Bräuer, Matze, Peter, Oleg, Oxx Beuter, Remel & Chressen, Dimi, Chiqui, Max & Malte, Seydi, Migo, and all those who I've forgotten. Thank you to Jarka Kubsova for the idea and for your help writing this book. You've had to learn half of a dentistry degree syllabus to truly understand what it's all about, and from the very beginning you've understood exactly what my goal is and what challenges would crop up. I'll never forget all the work we've done together. Thank you to my whole team at DNA Health & Aesthetics—I couldn't do any of this without you. You're the best team. I'd also like to thank my Juicery team. Thank you to my first teacher Dr. Manfred Wolf, who threw me in at the deep end and gave me the best possible basic surgical training. I will never forget. Thank you to my mentor in functional medicine and healing, Dietrich Klinghardt. I told you at the time that I would change conventional dentistry, and you told me that we are only strong when we work in a team. Thanks to my mentor and good friend Dr. Ulrich Volz, who taught me everything about ceramic implantology and much more. We are both on the same mission to change the world for the better.

I'd like to say a special thanks to my wife, Steffi, who always has my back and who has supported me for fifteen years, despite or maybe because of my hunger for extremes. You are always by my side and put everything into caring for me and our boys. To all the mothers out there: I truly appreciate the job you do 24/7 and would never be able to do it myself. You should be *proud*. I'd like to end my acknowledg-ments on this note: I want to stress that we are only strong as a *team* and that ultimately, it's important to surround ourselves with the right people who do not pull us down, but encourage us in what we do.

# NOTES

All websites listed were last consulted on November 30, 2018.

## Introduction

1. "WM 1958: Brasilien Wird Zur Fussball-Weltmacht," Deutscher
   Fussball-Bund, "News," https://www.dfb.de/news/detail/wm-1958
   -brasilien-wird-zur-fussball-weltmacht-21742.

## Chapter 1: Teeth and Microbiology

1. "Darmbakterien: Wie Sie Unser Gehirn Und Unsere Stimmung
   Beeinflussen," Magazin Wissen, Braineffect (website), https://www
   .brain-effect.com/magazin/darm-gehirn.
2. Jakob Simmank, "Da lebt was in Ihnen!" *Zeit Online*, July 11, 2017,
   http://www.zeit.de/wissen/2017-05/mikrobiom-bakterien-menschen
   -krankheit-forschung.
3. Joachim Klimek, *Speichel & Mundgesundheit: Ein Skript für Studenten
   zur Examensvorbereitung*, October 2014, http://fachschaft-zahnmedizin
   .de/wp-content/uploads/2012/10/ StuDent_Skript_Okt_2014-Speichel
   _Mundgesundheit.pdf.
4. "Bakterien der Mundflora Mögliche Ursache von CED," *Pharmazeutische
   Zeitung*, October 27, 2017, https://www.pharmazeutische-zeitung.de
   /index.php?id=72432.
5. "Bakterien im Mund: Ursache für Arteriosklerose?" *ZWP Online*,
   "Wissenschaft und Forschung," August 2, 2018, https://www.zwp
   -online.info/zwpnews/dental-news/wissenschaft-und-forschung
   /bakterien-mund-arteriosklerose.
6. Nancy Weiland-Bräuer et al., "Highly Effective Inhibition of Biofilm
   Formation by the First Metagenome-Derived Al-2 Quenching Enzyme,"
   *Frontiers in Microbiology* (July 2016), https://doi.org/10.3389/fmicb
   .2016.01098.
7. Wolfgang Buchalla, "Multitalent Speichel: Bekanntes und Neues zu
   Zusammensetzung und Fuktion," *Deutsche Zahnärztliche Zeitschrift* 67,
   no. 7 (2012): 438–46, http://doi.org/10.5167/uzh-73299.

8. Nicolas Dutzan et al., "On-Going Mechanical Damage from Mastication Drives Homeostatic Th17 Cell Responses at the Oral Barrier," *Immunity* 46, no. 1 (2017): 133–47, http://doi.org/10.1016/j.immuni.2016.12.010.

9. Federation of American Societies for Experimental Biology, "With Synthetic Mucus, Researchers Take Aim at Antibiotic Resistance," ScienceDaily, April 25, 2017, https://www.sciencedaily.com/releases/2017/04/170425175043.htm.

10. Hendrik Meyer-Lückel, Sebastian Paris, and Kim R. Ekstrand, eds., *Karies: Wissenschaft und Klinische Praxis* (Stuttgart, DE: Thieme, 2012), 162.

11. Meyer-Lückel, Paris, and Ekstrand, eds., *Karies*, 172.

12. Meyer-Lückel, Paris, and Ekstrand, eds., *Karies*, 162.

13. Philip Marsh and Michael V. Martin, *Orale Mikrobiologie: 60 Tabellen* (Stuttgart, DE: Thieme, 2003), 110.

14. "Röntgen beim Zahnarzt enthüllt Vitamin-D-Mangel," *ZWP Online*, "Wissenschaft und Forschung," January 15, 2018, https://www.zwp-online.info/zwpnews/dental-news/wissenschaft-und-forschung/roentgen-beim-zahnarzt-enthuellt-vitamin-d-mangel.

## Chapter 2: Teeth and the Immune System

1. Robert Kulacz and Thomas E. Levy, *The Roots of Disease: Connecting Dentistry and Medicine* (Bloomington, IN: Xlibris, 2002), 79.

2. Kulacz and Levy, *The Roots of Disease*, 43.

3. José F. Siqueira, Milton De Uzeda, and Maria Evangelina F. Fonseca, "A Scanning Electron Microscopic Evaluation of In Vitro Dentinal Tubules Penetration by Selected Anaerobic Bacteria," *Journal of Endodontics* 22, no. 6 (1996): 308–10, http://doi.org/10.1016/S0099-2399(96)80265-2; N. Richardson et al., "Microflora in Teeth Associated with Apical Periodontitis: A Methodological Observational Study Comparing Two Protocols and Three Microscopy Techniques," *International Endodontic Journal* 42, no. 10 (2009): 908–21.

4. A lot of researchers today prefer the expression fatty degenerative osteonecrosis jawbone (FDOJ). In the literature, you will also find the differential diagnosis of chronic ischemic bone disease (CIBD).

5. Johann Lechner, J. E. Bouqout, and Volker von Baehr, *Histologie und Immunologie der kavitätenbildenden Osteolysen des Kieferknochens* (Furth, DE: MDV Maristen, 2015).

6. Steven Lin, *Mundum Gesund: Die Richtige Ernahrung fur Zahne und Immunsystem*, trans. Elisabeth Liebl (Munich, DE: Scorpio Verlag, 2018), 48.

7. Lin, *Mundum Gesund*, trans. Elisabeth Liebl.

8. "Neue Forschung zur Komposit-Toxikologie," *ZM Online*, "Archiv," May 16, 2011, https://www.zm-online.de/archiv/2011/10/titel/neue -forschung-zur-komposit-toxikologie.

9. James C. Pendergrass and Boyd E. Haley, "Mercury EDTA Complex Specifically Blocks Brain-Tubulin-GTP Interactions: Similarity to Observations in Alzheimer's Disease," in *Status Quo and Perspectives of Amalgam and Other Dental Materials*, eds. L. T. Friberg and G. N. Schrauzer (Stuttgart, DE: Thieme, 1995), 98–105; James C. Pendergrass and Boyd E. Haley, "Inhibition of Brain Tubulin-Guanosine 5'-Triphosphate Interactions by Mercury: Similarity to Observations in Alzheimer's Diseased Brain," *Metal Ions in Biological Systems* 34 (1997): 461–78.

10. At the Bieger Laboratory in Munich (http://www.milab.de), the LTT method was used to examine over 1,000 people who were clinically suspected to have a hypersensitivity to prosthetic dental materials. The second most common allergen was gold (12 percent), ahead of mercury (10 percent), and palladium (6 percent).

11. Jenny A. Stejskal and Vera D. M. Stejskal, "The Role of Metals in Autoimmunity and the Link to Neuroendocrinology," *Neuroendocrinology Letters* 20, no. 6 (1999): 351–64.

12. D. Weingart et al., "Titanium Deposition in Regional Lymph Nodes After Insertion of Titanium Screw Implants in Maxillofacial Region," *International Journal of Oral and Maxillofacial Surgery* 23, no. 6, (1994): 450–52, http://doi.org/10.1016/0278-2391(95)90202-3.

13. H. Viranen et al., "Interaction of Mobile Phones with Superficial Passive Metallic Implants," *Physics in Medicine and Biology* 50, no. 11 (2005): 268–700, http://doi.org/10.1088/0031-9155/50/11/017.

## Chapter 3: Teeth and Chronic Disease

1. "Bakterien im Mund: Ursache für Arteriosklerose?" *ZWP Online*, "Wissenschaft und Forschung," August 2, 2018, https://www.zwp -online.info/zwpnews/dental-news/wissenschaft-und-forschung /bakterien-mund-arteriosklerose.

2. Lei Chen et al., "Association of Periodontal Parameters with Metabolic Level and Systemic Inflammatory Markers in Patients with Type 2 Diabetes," *Journal of Periodontology* 81, no. 3 (March 2010): https://doi .org/10.1902/jop.2009.090544.

3. Eike Fittig, Johannes Schweizer, and Udo Rudolph, "Lebenszufriedenheit bei Chronischen Erkrankungen: Zur Bedeutung

von Depressivität, Krankheitsverarbeitung und Sozialer Unterstützung,"
*Zeitschrift für Gesundheitspsychologie* 15, no. 1 (2007): 23–31, https://
doi.org/10.1026/0943-8149.15.1.23.

4. Cinthya Gomes et al., "Increased Root Canal Endotoxin Levels Are
Associated with Chronic Apical Periodontitis, Increased Oxidative
and Nitrosative Stress, Major Depression, Severity of Depression, and
a Lowered Quality of Life," *Molecular Neurobiology* 55, no. 4 (2018):
2814–27, http://doi.org/10.1007/s12035-017-0545-z.

5. "Mundgesundheit Beeinflusst Fruchtbarkeit," Zahnarztnachrichten,
Deutsche Zahnarzt Auskunft.de (website), June 25, 2014, http://www
.deutsche-zahnarztauskunft.de/zahnaerzte/zahnarztnachrichten
/singleview/?tx_ttnews[tt_news]=16327&cHash=ec531c0a574ab
354a0baec25eb95b945.

6. H Viranen et al., "Interaction of Mobile Phones with Superficial Passive
Metallic Implants," *Physics in Medicine and Biology* 50, no. 11 (2005):
2689–700, http://doi.org/10.1088/0031-9155/50/11/017.

7. Ingar Olsen and Sim K. Singhrao, "Can Oral Infection Be a Risk Factor
for Alzheimer's Disease?" *Journal of Oral Microbiology* 7 (2015): 29143,
http://doi.org/10.3402/jom.v7.29143.

8. Julie Lucifora et al., "Specific and Nonhepatotoxic Degradation of
Nuclear Hepatitis B Virus cccDNA," *Science* 343, no. 6176 (March 2014):
1221–8, http://doi.org/10.1126/science.1243462; Monika Julia Wolf et
al., "Metabolic Activation of Intrahepatic CD8+ T Cells and NKT Cells
Causes Nonalcoholic Steatohepatitis and Liver Cancer via Cross-Talk with
Hepatocytes," *Cancer Cell* 26, no. 4 (October 2014): 549–64, https://doi
.org/10.1016/j.ccell.2014.09.003; Monika Julia Wolf et al., "Endothelial CCR2
Signaling Induced by Colon Carcinoma Cells Enables Extravasation via
the JAK2-Stat5 and p38MAPK Pathway," *Cancer Cell* 22, no. 1 (July 2012):
91–105; Johannes Haybaeck et al., "A Lymphotoxin-Driven Pathway to
Hepatocellular Carcinoma," *Cancer Cell* 16, no.4 (October 2009): 295–308.

## Chapter 4: Get Healthy and Stay Healthy with Biological Dentistry

1. Lois Y. Matsuoka et al., "Sunscreens Suppress Cutaneous Vitamin $D_3$
Synthesis," *Journal of Clinical Endocrinology and Metabolism* 64, no. 6
(1987): 1165–68, http://doi.org/10.1210/jcem-64-6-1165.

2. Thomas L. Clemens et al., "Increased Skin Pigment Reduces the
Capacity of Skin to Synthesise Vitamin $D_3$," *Lancet* 319, no. 8263 (1982):
74–76, http://doi.org/10.1016/S0140-6736(82)90214-8.

3. John J. Cannell, William B. Grant, and Michael F. Holick, "Vitamin D and Inflammation," *Dermato-Endocrinology* 6, no. 1 (2014): e983401, http://doi.org/10.4161/19381980.2014.983401.

4. Ulrike Schulze-Späte et al., "Systemic Vitamin D Supplementation and Local Bone Formation after Maxillary Sinus Augmentation: A Randomized, Double-Blind, Placebo-Controlled Clinical Investigation," *Clinical Oral Implants Research* 27, no. 6 (2016): 701–06, http://doi.org/10.1111/clr.12641; Simon Spedding, "Vitamin D and Depression: A Systematic Review and Meta-Analysis Comparing Studies with and without Biological Flaws," *Nutrients* 6, no. 4 (2014): 1501–18, http://doi.org/10.3390/nu6041501.

5. Anne Marie Uwitonze and Mohammed Razzaque, "Role of Magnesium in Vitamin D Activation and Function," *Journal of the American Osteopathic Association* 118, no. 3 (2018): 181–89, http://doi.org/10.7556/jaoa.2018.037.

6. Steven Lin, *The Dental Diet: The Surprising Link Between Your Teeth, Real Food, and Life-Changing Natural Health* (London: Hay House, 2018), 123.

7. *Fünfte Deutsche Mundgesundheitsstudie (DMS V): Kurzfassung* (Institut der Deutschen Zahnärzte, 2016), https://www.bzaek.de/fileadmin/PDFs/dms/Zusammenfassung_DMS_V.pdf.

8. Corinna Flemming, "Anzahl der Zähne Bestimmt, wie Alt Wir Werden," *ZWP Online*, "Wissenschaft und Forschung," February 3, 2018, https://www.zwp-online.info/zwpnews/dental-news/wissenschaft-und-forschung/anzahl-der-zaehne-bestimmt-wie-alt-wir-werden.

# INDEX

nervus trigeminus. *See* trigeminal nerve
neuralgia-inducing cavitational
	osteonecroses. *See* NICOs
	(neuralgia-inducing cavitational
	osteonecroses)
neural therapy, 83, 87
neuromodulatory triggers, 91
neurotransmitters
	cultivation of, by bacteria, 12
	in the gut, 152–55
	obtaining profile of, 153
nickel, in amalgam fillings, 71
NICOs (neuralgia-inducing
	cavitational osteonecroses)
	causes of, 61–64
	treatment of, 64–67, 124–26
noradrenaline
	methylation concerns, 75
	in stress response, 66, 92
	vitamin C for production and
		regeneration of, 90, 150
nutrient deficiencies
	effects on tooth pulp, 35
	in the elderly, 162
	healing process impeded by, 126
	jaw malformations linked to, 66–67
	leaky gut syndrome and, 142
	overview, 147–150
	sensitive teeth from, 165
nutrient timing, 134
nutrition
	connection to jaw malformations,
		66–67
	for the elderly, 162
	healing power of, 126–28
	importance during recovery from
		illness, 49
	importance to detoxification, 75,
		76, 77
	pre-operative concerns, 126
	Price, Weston research, 33–36, 66–67
	*See also* micronutrients

nutritional toxins, 128, 140
nutrition plans. *See* food
	recommendations
nuts, recommended types, 130

obesity, link to diseases of the mouth,
	103–4
odontoblasts, 52, *54*
oil pulling, 18, 164
omega-3 fatty acids, 136–37, 153
opportunistic bacteria, 9
	*See also* bacteria
oral health
	iatrogenic factors in dental
		problems, 36–41
	importance of nutrition, 33–36
	need for balance among
		microorganisms, 9–10
oral hygiene
	for children, 160–61
	for the elderly, 161–63
	frequently asked questions, 163–66
	historical approaches, 27–28
	insufficiency of, 3
	Price, Weston research, 34
	professional cleanings, 162, 165
	receding gums from improper
		technique, 43
oral microbia
	complexity of, 28
	discovery of, 6–10
	filling materials and, 39–41
	food recommendations, 150–52
	homeostasis in, 25–26
	metabolism of sugars, 30–33
	pH levels and, 23–24
organic foods, 135, 145
osteolyses, 62

pain
	from death of tooth, 51
	fear of, 166

# ABOUT THE AUTHOR

D r. Dominik Nischwitz is a dentist and naturopath, a world specialist in biological dentistry and ceramic implants, and the president of the International Society of Metal Free Implantology (ISMI). In 2015, Dr. Nischwitz cofounded DNA Health and Aesthetics, Center for Biological Dentistry with his father in Tübingen, Germany. Dr. Nischwitz has exclusively used ceramic implants since 2013, placing more than 3,000 to date. A pioneer in the field of holistic odontology, Dr. Nischwitz regularly gives lectures around the world. He trains traditional dentists in biological dentistry and believes that all health starts in the mouth.